THE MARATHON WE LIVE:
Training for a Personal Best in Life with Type 1 Diabetes

Courtney J. Duckworth

DEDICATION

This book is dedicated to those who ran this race before us, especially Linda.

CONTENTS

Author's Note..vii

Introduction: The Starting Line................................1

Part I: Ready. Set. Wait...Where am I Going? And Why? The *What* and the *Want*..................................21

Part II: Learning (and Relearning) About the Task at Hand..49

Part III: Forming (and Reforming) Strategies................75

Part IV: Building Endurance to Go the Distance.............97

A Personal Best..133

Resources..135

Endnotes...147

Bibliography...153

Acknowledgments..157

AUTHOR'S NOTE

First things first: you don't have to be a marathon runner to read this book. Training for marathons is not an experience many people get to have…or want to have for that matter. And that's totally okay. If the only running you have done is catching the morning bus, this book is for you. If you're a 100-mile ultramarathoner, this book is also for you.

Now that we covered who you *don't* have to be, here's who you *do* have to be: someone who wants to be better in his or her type 1 diabetes (T1D) management. I have been one of these people since I was diagnosed at the age of ten. I will always be one of these people. 14 years later and I still don't have diabetes "figured out" (no one really does), but every day I work to be better.

Growing up, I had little direction in my management nor consistency in my control. My results were often disappointing, yet simply "trying harder" didn't get me very far. After bursts of temporary changes, I ended up overwhelmed, discouraged, and right back to where I started. Those years were filled with unnecessary frustration, feelings of guilt, and lost benefits to my health. Worst of all, I felt alone in what I was experiencing…other people with T1D looked so healthy. Surely they were not struggling like I was.

If I could go back to my teenage self as she grappled with these thoughts, I would tell her this:

1) You're not alone. Nobody is in range 100% of the time. In fact, ~85% of teens and young adults similarly struggle to reach treatment goals recommended by the American Diabetes Association.[1]

2) Progress > Perfection. Trust the process...focusing on small, daily victories in management will lead to better control over time. Really, small decisions add up.

Even after years of working on this project, I am regularly reminded to reflect on these lessons for peace of mind and motivation. The mission of this book is to provide readers with similar comfort and inspiration to take positive steps in their care. If this book accomplishes that—even for just one person—every experience behind these words will have been worth it.

Medical Disclaimer: I am not a doctor (yet). The purpose of this book is to promote healthy living with T1D and share what has been helpful in my personal care. Before making changes to your medical regimen, it is always best to consult with a doctor or certified diabetes educator.

INTRODUCTION

THE STARTING LINE

I believe everything happens for a reason. The experiences we have and the people we meet are not accidents. Case in point: my introduction to life with T1D. A few years before I was diagnosed, my family received a letter in the mail from a girl named Caity. Caity was six years old like me and lived in Washington state about 2,800 miles away from our home near Washington, D.C.

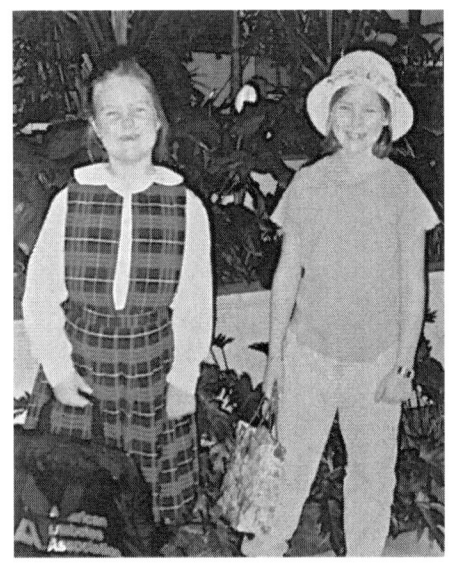

Caity (right) and me (left) as first graders in 1999.

We were alike in many ways...except for needles. Caity had to endure four shots a day. She also pricked her fingers to test her blood sugar....even more than she had to take shots. Kids like me dreaded their annual flu shots. Caity's bravery was beyond anything I could fathom.

The purpose of Caity's letter was twofold. One, to raise awareness for T1D. It certainly accomplished that. Two, to gain support for Petition for a Cure. The petition would raise awareness at the level of policy makers who could increase funding. More funding, more research. More research, maybe fewer shots for Caity and millions of other people with T1D.

For months, I collected signatures from everyone I knew, and then sent them to Caity. With her untiring initiative and help from others, she collected over 2.3 million signatures and was able to present the petition to lawmakers in Washington, D.C. We met briefly in person during her visit and kept in loose contact over the years until a phone call from my mother to hers reconnected us. The message: I had also been diagnosed with T1D.

I was nine years old when I temporarily lost vision and hearing during a school church service. In that moment, for some inexplicable reason, I wasn't all that afraid. Within the five or so minutes of no sight nor sound, I had already planned how to continue the most important activity in my life: figure skating. I had seen the 1970s movie *Ice Castles* and reasoned if Lynn-Holly Johnson could skate without vision, so could I. Everything would be okay.

While contemplating the other details of my new life, a loud ringing noise entered my ears. Sounds slowly returned. My vision progressed to seeing lights and shadows. A few minutes later, I felt relatively fine. So much for my skating career as Lynn-Holly Johnson. But what had just happened?

At the time, my sister and I were new students at a religious school and going to church was a weekly occurrence. I was kneeling in a church pew on a Wednesday morning when the episode occurred. Right after the service, I went straight to the school nurse. She didn't believe me.

"So you had a holy vision or something? Well even if you are a saint one day, I'm not letting you go home early." Little did she know that over the next four years, she would be seeing me quite a bit more. And not for "holy visions."

My pediatrician decided to wait and see if anything happened again. Nothing did. I was a little dizzy upon standing from time to time, but didn't think twice about it. Aside from the episode at church, the only odd thing in the weeks before my diagnosis was a feeling. I remember describing it to my dad as "feeling like there was something missing." Looking back now, that seems pretty ominous.

A few weeks later during routine blood work for my ten-year checkup, results picked up an abnormally high blood sugar. Despite my mother and me trying to convince the doctors they were wrong, I was diagnosed with T1D on my tenth birthday…which falls right before Halloween. Definitely not the ideal time for a diagnosis. Thus began a mission to prove (mostly to myself) that despite T1D, I could accomplish anything. In those days, "anything" consisted of doing well in school and reaching the highest levels of competitive figure skating.

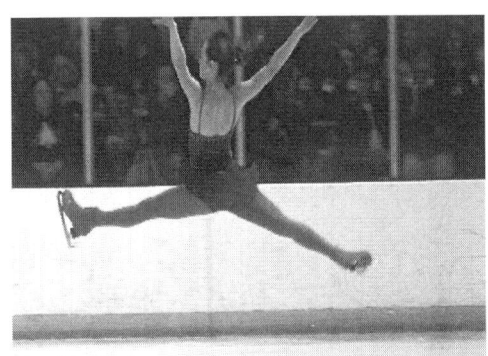

Flying high during my favorite program, "Ave Maria," in high school.

After the initial shock of learning new management skills and fitting them into my daily routine, I found life with T1D to be complicated, but manageable. The only time I was truly inconvenienced was during low blood sugars. Those were scary. They removed me from school, sports, and friends. They made me feel different. A little high though, and I could function just fine. Given the choice of risking low blood sugars or being "safe" a little high, I would usually choose the latter.

Every three months, A1Cs served as reminders of the concrete consequences to what seemed like harmless choices. I would focus harder on management for a while, but wouldn't see consistent improvement in my blood sugars and become discouraged. Eventually, my fear-driven motivation would dissipate and I would fall back into the same mindset and management habits.

I cared. I tried to practice a healthy lifestyle. I was interested in learning as much as possible about the human body (an interest that would eventually lead to a career in medicine), but didn't apply what I was learning and let T1D come second to other, more immediate tasks. As a result, I didn't have the best control. I held onto the vague idea that one day, a switch would flip and my control would magically fall into place. This pattern went on for nearly a decade.

It was one sentence that finally made it click: "That felt like running an 8:45 mile when you're expecting a 7:15."

For that sentence to make any sense at all, let me provide some background...

I was a running-crazed 20 year old when I said those words to my mom. It was after a particularly disappointing endocrinology appointment. My A1C was 8.9%. For a decade of living with T1D, that's really not fantastic. It was embarrassing that I hadn't figured out how to have tighter control. I had managed to become good at other things in life. Why not T1D?

Leading up to the appointment, I had run three marathons to successfully qualify for the Boston Marathon. But I had not grown up as a runner. Or even liking to run for that matter. The most running I ever did was a few laps around the parking lot as a warmup for skating. And I did them begrudgingly. When there were hurdles in P.E. class, forget it! I faked a low blood sugar.

The obsession with running and Boston started during spring break my sophomore year at the College of William and Mary when my friend, Thomas, brought up bucket lists. Some of the items on my list included:

> Travel to all 7 continents
> Try out for the Washington Capitals Red Rockers
> Speak at the Friends for Life Conference in Orlando
> Find an arrowhead
> Run a marathon
> Become a doctor
> Start a college scholarship for students with T1D
> Take mom to see the *Ellen Show*

Turns out, Thomas shared one of these items: run a marathon.* Possibly out of boredom, he suggested something crazy…that we should do it…and start our training right there on the spot. Not wanting to seem tentative, I went along with it. At the time, I didn't think he was actually being serious.

We knew absolutely nothing about running marathons. So there we were in my kitchen, searching for training plans online. Anything from "The Lazy Girl's Guide to Marathon Running" to expert Hal Higdon's racing tips. Our plan was more like "The Lazy Higdon's Guide to Marathon Running" with an averaged difficulty of the plans we found. We figured we could adjust it as needed. All we wanted was to finish a race.

---

* Other items in common included: become a doctor and travel to all seven continents. Not surprisingly, he had no ambition of becoming a professional cheerleader.

We decided on a 16-week training plan with four runs each week. Long runs on Saturdays, two days of cross-training, and rest on Sundays. In typical Type A fashion, I made a spreadsheet with boxes to check off all 112 days before the race. That way, we were held accountable for completing runs and could have confidence in our preparation when the time came for the full 26.2 miles.

We chose an early summer race in Lake Placid and BOOM...just like that, in less than an hour, we were ready to run our first marathon. Then reality hit...how was I supposed to run for 3-4 hours *and* keep stable blood sugars? What would I eat? What if I went low?!

Sensing my hesitation, Thomas gave me the reassurance I'm sure he thought any woman would want to hear. "If Oprah can run a marathon, so can we." Oprah...a marathon? Really? More importantly, how did Thomas know that?

Sure enough, Oprah had run the Marine Corps Marathon in 1994. By doing so, she inspired a whole new wave of marathon runners who had never stepped foot on pavement, but had what it takes to go the distance. So maybe it was possible. Plus, I knew other people with T1D had competed in extreme sports—marathons, triathlons, mountain climbing. If they could do it, there *was* a way. I would just have to find it.

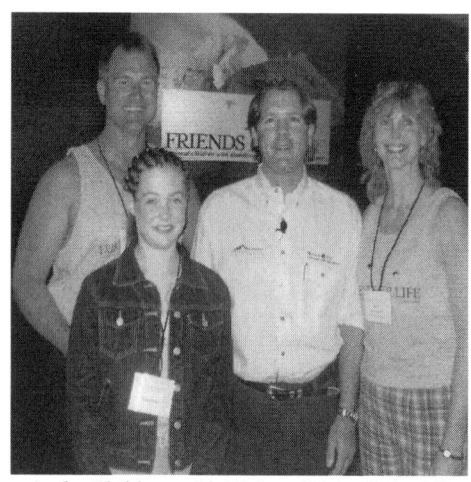

At the Children with Diabetes' Friends for Life Conference in 2004, my family and I got to meet Will Cross who successfully climbed Mt. Everest with T1D. In 2017, I had the opportunity to attend the same conference as a speaker!

When we got back to school, training officially began. The lack of stopping in running was a completely foreign concept. "Short" runs of five miles seemed exceedingly difficult. My legs felt pain that was completely unlike that of skating and it took awhile to build endurance. Most of all, the idea of no designated stopping to test my blood sugar made me uneasy. A loud voice in my head always questioned what my blood sugars were doing and if I was really feeling my lows. Had I taken too much insulin? Not enough insulin? It all seemed like a big, risky experiment.

In reality, it was. I had no record of what was working on runs and what was not. When I would finish a long run in range, it was 90% luck and 10% of what I happened to remember from past runs. I was wasting valuable clues to which combinations of insulin, food, and timing worked best.

The pinnacle of my experimentation came about two months into training on a Saturday morning around 6:30 a.m. Thomas and I usually did long runs together so he could hold my extra glucose. Up to that point, I had never needed to use it and figured I would be just fine going solo.

Per usual, I didn't pay too much attention to food or bolus insulin. I ate, reduced my insulin by a random amount that seemed right, and decided to try something new: take my long-acting basal insulin before the run instead of after. Why I tried something new the day I was running alone is beyond me...not a smart move (please don't try this at home!).

The run started down Colonial Parkway leading to a spot every student called "Jamestown Beach." A really pretty run and not too much traffic. But about four miles in, I started feeling lightheaded and tested—53 mg/dL (2.9 mmol/L). I had a whole roll of glucose tabs. Waited 20 minutes—45 mg/dL (2.5 mmol/L)...had another roll of glucose tabs. Waited 20 minutes—35 mg/dL (1.9 mmol/L) and officially out of glucose. I needed help, but no cars had passed by all morning. And not a soul in sight.

I tried calling all my close friends, but of course no one was up that early on a Saturday in college. My last and only resort was 9-1-1.

"9-1-1, what's your emergency?"

Through tears (also new at the whole 9-1-1 thing), I said, "Hi, my name is Courtney Duckworth. I am 19 years old and have type 1 diabetes. My blood sugar is low and dropping and I ran out of glucose. I'm sitting on the side of the road by Jamestown Beach."

"Do you see a ferry?"

"There are no ferries here."

"Then you're not at Jamestown Beach."

"I took a right down Colonial Parkway and ran four miles from William and Mary's campus. Where does that put me?"

"I don't know, but we can't send a dispatch team until we know your exact location."

I started to panic. My emergency help was no help at all or didn't know how to operate GPS (either way, she was in the wrong profession). I wasn't wearing a medical ID so even if someone were to find me, they would have no idea how to treat my emergency. I was convinced I would die at what was apparently not Jamestown Beach.

While still on the phone with 9-1-1, a car parked on the side of the road. A dad with two young sons and a kite got out. It was a miracle. With all of my uncoordinated, low-blood-sugar effort, I ran over and asked for a ride back to campus. My dispatcher was beside herself.

"What are you doing?"

"Getting REAL help. Bye!"

Like any good dad to young kids, the man had juice boxes and snacks in his car. They probably saved my life.

That incident was a huge wake up call. I needed a better system. From that day on, I kept a log of what I tried and the results. Item 1: DO NOT take full basal dose right before a run. From there, things got a little more detailed: time of day, mileage, carbs, insulin, and starting and ending blood sugars.

Pretty soon, I started finding strategies that worked and wasn't just getting by on luck. I could be more certain that what I did was safe and effective. Why? Because it had been before. As I got more confident that I would have stable blood sugars, that loud, nagging voice in my head started to quiet down. Just like skating had been, running became a sort of escape from everyday life and T1D. With running came *freedom*. And when I started to improve and complete progressively longer runs, I got really addicted. I had no idea how fast I was, but could run without stopping for a long time and loved it. It felt like I was proving myself wrong and even other people who tried to convince me after the Jamestown Beach incident that running a marathon with T1D would be too dangerous.

Of course, there was still an air of uncertainty. My longest run had been 18 miles. Eight miles and about an hour less than a full marathon. Those of you with T1D know—a lot can happen to blood sugars during an hour of vigorous exercise. I was cautiously optimistic. I believed beyond doubt that with stable blood sugars, I could do *anything*, including cross the finish line.[†]

The race started and ended in downtown Lake Placid. Two 13.1-mile loops through the Adirondack Mountains. As soon as the race began, I felt at peace. I had put in all the hard work. Now only a few hours separated me from crossing

---

[†] Note the contrast between previous thinking of being able to do anything *despite* T1D versus being able to do anything by working *with* T1D.

an item off my bucket list. Using the routine that had worked best in training, my blood sugar stayed stable into mile 10….and then 15…and then 20.

The biggest physical challenge was "hitting the wall" around mile 21. It's at this point in a marathon when runners are most tempted to give up. Glycogen (the body's stored form of glucose) depots are exhausted. The legs get heavy. Breathing becomes difficult. The body reaches maximum physical exhaustion. Training brings runners to that point, but going all the way takes digging a little deeper. And I had plenty to keep me going—the thought of crossing the finish line within the hour, the pride of representing all people with T1D, and proving that running a marathon wasn't "too dangerous"…that it *was* possible. It was mind over matter. Each step was taking me closer.

Before I knew it, my name was being announced to the crowd as I crossed the finish line and received a medal. I was so overjoyed that I even re-ran the last stretch of the race with Thomas. And as we waited for our final times to be posted, we did what any responsible runners would do after a big race—refueled with Ben & Jerry's Banana Peanut Butter Greek Frozen Yogurt.

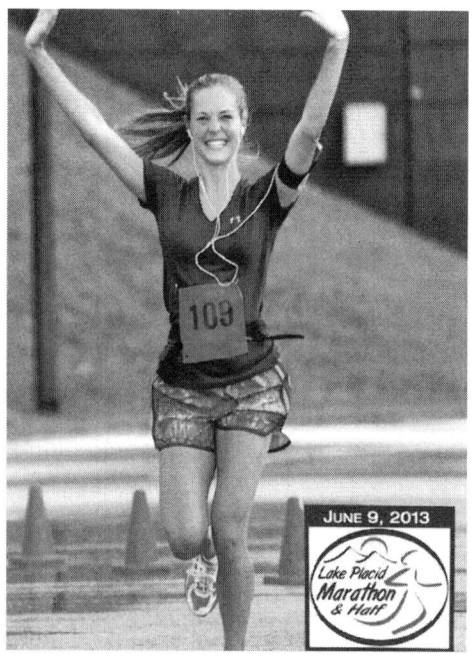

All smiles on the final stretch of the Lake Placid Marathon!

With frozen yogurt in hand, we looked up times of Boston Marathon champions and qualifying times for fun—3:35:00 for women and 3:05:00 for men our age. We didn't have a reference for exactly how fast that was, but estimated our times had been around 4:00:00 in comparison.

Then we saw our actual times. I had run a 3:38:39. Enough to win the 20-and-under age group! But what *really* excited me was how close it was to a Boston qualifying time. I had never trained for speed and knew with proper training, I could compete in Boston.

Instead of going home and crossing "run a marathon" off my bucket list, I crossed out "a" and inserted two words…"the Boston." Two little words that would lead to thousands of miles worth of training.

To shave four minutes off my time, each mile would have to be about 10 seconds faster. Seemed easy enough…but how? The first step was picking a course with flatter terrain. Growing up in northern VA, I had heard good things about the Marine Corps Marathon (MCM). That year, the race was on my 20th birthday…also the 10th anniversary of my T1D diagnosis. Not to mention, it was Oprah's race of choice back in 1994. The MCM would be ideal.

Next, the harder part: becoming a faster runner. Above all else, I needed to be aware of my pace, so I bought a running watch with GPS. Next, I needed to do some research. In elite running, speed is the name of the game. How did other distance runners go about training for speed? What skills did I need to build?

Using these new tools, research, and what I had learned from Lake Placid, I upgraded "The Lazy Higdon's Guide to Marathon Running" to a training plan that was a little more sophisticated. Now it included specific strength and speed exercises to be performed on certain days of the week. I was more thoughtful about warming up and cooling down. I monitored nutrition—what I ate before, during, and after runs as well as what I ate on days when I wasn't running at all. And of course, I focused on strategies for tighter blood sugar control, which changed as my body became more adapted to running.

    I made another 16-week plan and then followed through one day at a time, tweaking strategies here and there as I continued trying new things and figuring out what worked best. Within about eight weeks of this new training regimen, I noticed a consistently faster pace. By the time of the MCM, my pace was around 7:30 min/mile on shorter runs and 7:55 min/mile on long runs. If I could stay around that pace, I would finish with a time of 3:27:34. Well within Boston's qualifying standards.

    When it came time for the race, nearly every training run was complete. I had no injuries and up to that point in my life, I had never been in better shape. But on the day of the race, conditions were not in my favor. I woke up around 3 a.m. with a migraine and vomiting. When it came time to leave for the race, I was nauseous and severely dehydrated.

    On a regular day, I wouldn't have dreamed of running five miles like that, let alone 26.2 miles. But the race wasn't just about me—I was running for those with T1D and as a runner for the Diabetes Action Research and Education Foundation. Countless people had sponsored and supported me throughout training.

    One of those people was Linda, a woman who had also been a Tri Delta at the College of William and Mary and had grown up with T1D. When she contacted me, she had been living with T1D for 62 years. She reached out via email with the subject line reading, "The Marathon We Live." We bonded over stories of T1D experimentation. Balancing insulin and exercise. Trying to count carbs in mysterious dining hall foods. The uncertainty that comes with handling new situations in management.

Except Linda's version of "experimentation" was much more extreme. Our 48-year age gap proved to be an *eternity* in the world of T1D. When Linda was in college, T1D treatment and awareness were nowhere near what they are today. She dealt with primitive technology, rigid daily routines, and a terrifying level of uncertainty.

In the few decades after she was diagnosed, there was no at-home blood glucose testing. Instead, blood sugars were measured 3-4 times a year at the doctor's office. On a daily basis, she was only able to detect abnormally high blood sugars with urine tests. When it came to insulin, Linda took one shot of long-acting insulin in the morning and was prescribed certain foods to eat at specific times of the day. To make sure the serving size was correct, she meticulously weighed foods with a scale. Since there was no rapid-acting insulin, she had no flexibility in her diet, which made it difficult to coordinate meals with friends who could eat whatever and whenever they wanted.

With no meters to provide advanced warning for low blood sugars, she had many spells of unconsciousness. Teachers, friends, and peers *had* to know about her T1D to look for symptoms of low blood sugars before they became serious. Since some of these symptoms happen just by being nervous or a normal teenager (like sweatiness or irritability), there were probably a lot of frustrating discrepancies in predicting lows.

Despite these challenges, Linda had lived 62 years with T1D. She raised children, had a great job at NASA, and changed lives as an active member of the T1D community. Most notably, she never talked negatively about her experiences with T1D. She was grateful for the opportunity to live and her enthusiasm for each and every day was contagious.

Our exchanges lasted for a brief period of time until Linda passed away from cancer. I thought of her often during training runs and at the MCM, she fueled my motivation—if Linda could bravely pursue a limitless life with T1D in some of its earliest times of treatment, I could certainly find the bravery to run the MCM after a migraine...or at least try. I owed it to Linda. I owed it to everyone else. I owed it to myself. Boston was *our* mission.

Because getting sick delayed the departure from home, I was late to the starting line and missed my chorale—the group of runners who ran around the same pace. Instead, I started behind a large crowd of people doing the race for fun...and doing it very slowly. Mile after mile, I saw minutes being added to my time as I desperately tried to weave in and out of the crowd. By mile 12, the course started opening up and I *booked* it. If I could go that far without passing out, maybe just maybe I could run fast enough to make up for the additional time. Maybe I could still qualify for Boston. Approaching the end of the race, I knew it would be close.

My parents and Thomas were in the crowd and were tracking my location, pace, and finish time with their smartphones (isn't technology cool?!).

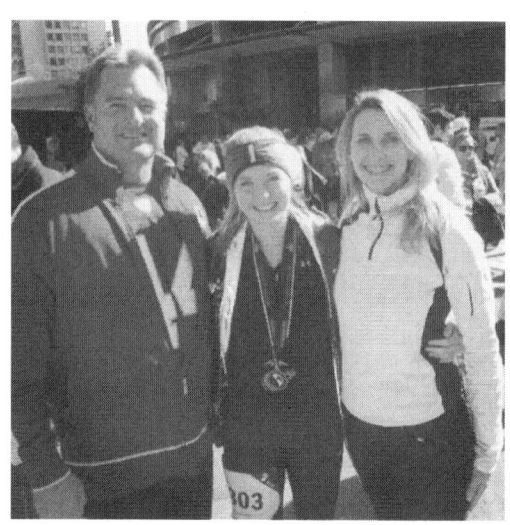

We were disappointed I did not qualify at the MCM, but relieved that I had finished the race.

Although they were relieved and surprised that I made it all the way to the end, the looks on their faces gave it away—my time hadn't been enough. 3:35:21. 21 seconds away from a qualifying time.

I was a little disappointed, but kept things in perspective. God had guided me to the race's finish. I hadn't passed out. My blood sugar was a little high, but no ketones. I thought, "Boston isn't meant to be *right now*, but that doesn't mean it's *never* meant to be." I could run as many races as my body would allow.

However, I didn't really want to run another marathon soon after the MCM. I was tired of training and tired of putting my body through the pain day after day after day. I wanted to be a regular college student again—one who could be flexible with workouts, have time with friends, and be able to sleep in on Saturday mornings. But fate had other plans, and so did Thomas.

"If you try just one more time, I'll run the race with you."

When someone selflessly volunteers to run hundreds of miles just to see you try one more time, it's pretty hard to say "no." He believed I could do it. Probably even more than I did.

One month later, we were back at it to train for the Columbia Marathon—a race held in South Carolina over the spring break of our junior year. I continued to learn with experience. How to run when there's a blizzard outside. How to run while nursing an injury. And how to tweak my insulin...this time with an insulin pump. Of course, just like before, finding the right strategies took a lot of trial-and-error. But this time, I knew to play it safe, and then slowly increase insulin as needed. Not the other way around.

Training for the MCM, I was confident I would qualify for Boston. Going into Columbia, I was much more grounded. Of course I trained to qualify, but so much was still out of my hands. I could only do the best with the conditions I was given. And conditions still weren't fantastic.

The day before the race, the infusion sets for my insulin pump weren't inserting correctly and I wasn't receiving any insulin. After carb-loading, this quickly turned into sky-high blood sugars and ketones. Luckily, I recognized what was happening and switched back to shots around 2 a.m. the morning of the race. With ketones cleared and an insulin pen in my fanny pack, Thomas and I made our way to the starting line. Beyond that speed bump, so many things went *right*. The weather was good, I didn't have a migraine, no crowds. I still had a fair shot.

For the first 18 miles, I kept up with the pacer who was estimated to finish at 3:30:00. Definitely within qualifying standards. But then I started to lose him and he ran out of sight. Around mile 23, the 3:35:00 pacer passed me, too. It didn't make sense according to the time on my running watch, but pacers don't lie, right?

For the next three miles, I felt like I was chasing the golden snitch from *Harry Potter*. That pacer represented my goal of Boston. All the miles, sweat, tears, experimentation...I would never forgive myself for letting him slip away.

On the final stretch, there we were: the 3:35:00 pacer and me...sprinting to catch up. As we got closer, I saw the official clock time: 3:30:00. The pacer had

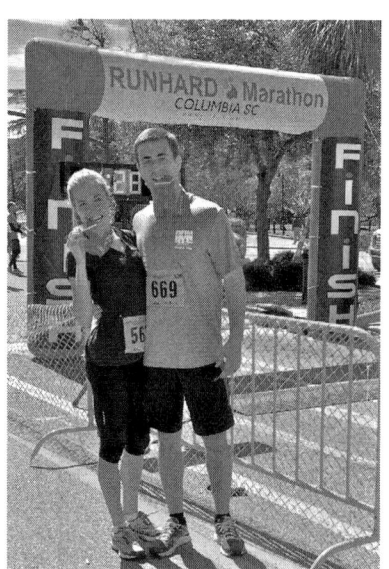

Thomas and me at the finish of the Columbia Marathon. Because he challenged me to another race, I qualified for Boston.

outpaced himself. I was going to qualify...with time to spare!

Reflecting on everything that went into that moment, the feeling was incredible. All of the pain, doubts, and sacrifices were worth it. Every race, I found ways to train better and it showed in my times...3:38:39, 3:35:21, and 3:30:48. Fast forward a year later and I would cross the Boston Marathon finish line in 3:25:53 (more on Boston's story in Part IV).

It's soon after qualifying at Columbia that my 8.9% A1C intersects.

There I was with top-notch technology, an awesome endocrinologist, a good amount of the basic physiological knowledge behind T1D management (I was premed for goodness sake!). I lived a healthy lifestyle, had the support of family and friends, and knew I was capable of better. So why couldn't I figure it out?

"That felt like running an 8:45 mile when you're expecting a 7:15."

Wait. "The Marathon We Live." Maybe Linda was onto something. What if living with T1D was like running marathons? Just like running, better results in T1D would require training. And why not apply the same approach that had already worked well with marathons?

After a lot of reflection (probably too much reflection) I broke down the four steps that had been essential in every race:

1) knowing the race I was training for and why;
2) creating a foundation of knowledge, and continuously building on it;
3) forming strategies based on knowledge, and tweaking them with experience; and
4) developing the mental endurance to maintain training over time.

Most importantly, I realized the "magic switch" I was relying on didn't exist. Better control wouldn't happen overnight. Instead, it would happen gradually in small steps.

To build my management skills, I started targeting what seemed like minute actions. Measuring food. Varying the times of my testing. Setting an alarm to change out my pump site. These small actions were like dominoes. Improvements in one area of care improved others, too. Taking time to carefully count carbs made me less likely to snack without a bolus. Testing after meals made me more inclined to time insulin correctly. Changing out my pump site every few days made me more attentive to changing out lancets.

While I didn't execute these little actions 100% all of the time, I applied a marathon-like mindset. It wasn't about being perfect, it was about being *better*. Doing my *best*. This mindset especially helped with out-of-range numbers. They were now just part of a much larger process. Not failures, but rather clues as to what worked in my care and what did not.

Over time, applying lessons from marathon training allowed for little changes to add up. My results weren't perfect and there were plenty of off-days, but my A1Cs gradually decreased. My blood sugars were more predictable and I gained greater confidence in my management. There was *direction*.

I felt "fine" a little high, but I felt *good* when I was in range…both physically and mentally. Being in range more often allowed me to excel in the activities that mattered most.

I noticed faster recovery after runs as my body had the insulin to use nutrients effectively. This contributed to a new personal best at the Boston Marathon. Additionally, better control boosted focus and flexibility in tasks outside of running, such as taking the required admission test for medical school and working as a clinical research fellow at the National Institutes of Health.

INTRODUCTION | 19

Taking a marathon approach in my care has also been a cornerstone in learning to manage T1D as a professional cheerleader (a part-time passion in addition to research and running). As a marathon runner and professional athlete, I have been blessed with the opportunity to speak on balancing sports with T1D at research summits, conferences, and camps for people with T1D.

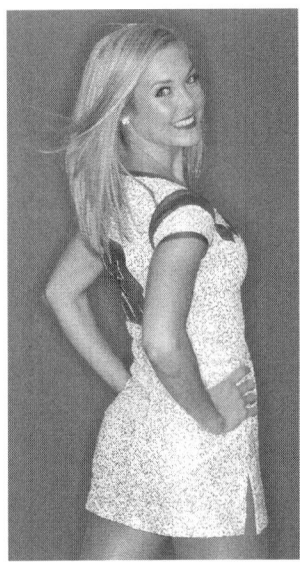
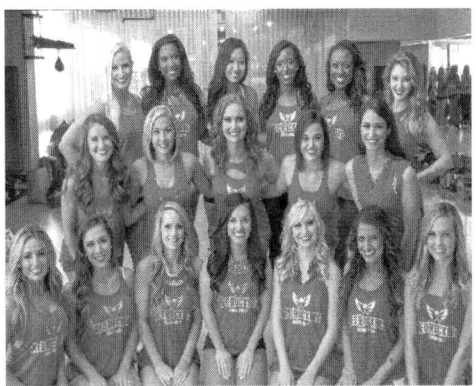

Being on the Red Rockers has brought about amazing opportunities and the chance to spread awareness for T1D! My teammates have become some of my greatest friends and always have my back. *Photos courtesy of the Washington Capitals and Ned Dishman.*

In the future as a medical student, doctor, and athlete, I know the stepwise approach laid out in this book will be essential to my success and ability to help other people.

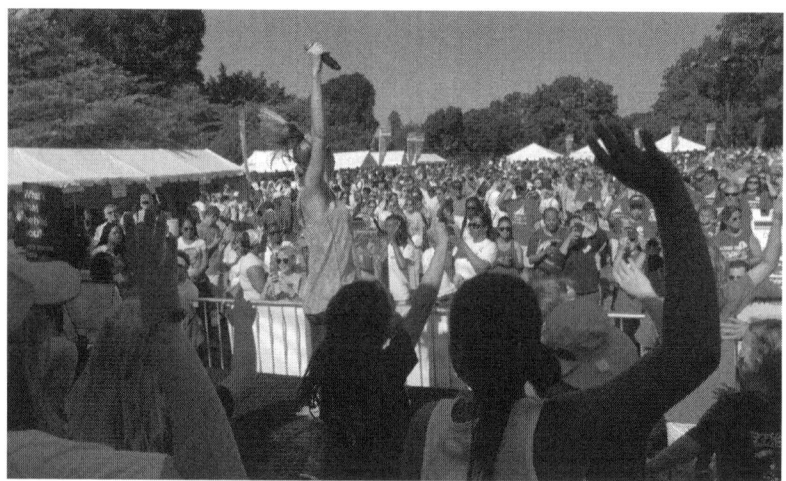

Leading the warm up at the JDRF OneWalk in Washington, D.C.

While practice doesn't necessarily "make perfect" (in T1D, there's no such thing!), training can make us better. And that's what this book is all about. By sharing the lessons that have shaped my management and positively influenced areas of life that extend far beyond T1D, it is my hope that others will be inspired to invest in one step today that will continue to pay off down the road….to reach for new personal bests right now and in the many miles yet to come.

With that said, let's run!

PART I

READY. SET. WAIT…WHERE AM I GOING? AND WHY? THE *WHAT* AND THE *WANT*

Without question, runners in training know two things at all times: *what* event they're training for and why they *want* to train in the first place. A 5K to work up to three consecutive miles. A ten-miler to raise money for a favorite charity. A half marathon for a new personal record. In my case, a full marathon to cross off a bucket list item.

In addition to big-picture motivators, runners also use smaller, daily incentives to stay on track. Eating peanut butter and an apple after a run. Time outside. A chance to get away. Bonding with friends. Accomplishing the workout for the day. Feeling strong, empowered, and relaxed.

Without knowing exactly *what* one is trying to accomplish, effective training is impossible. Without the pull from personalized big-picture and daily motivators—our *wants*—training won't last. In T1D, before we're ready to put in any work to improve our management, we have to know our *what* and our *wants*.

The *What*

As people with T1D, we hear the phrase "control" all the time. We're supposed to strive for it constantly, yet it can be difficult to know what we should be aiming for and how it translates to our daily care. What does "control" really mean?

In a nutshell, control refers to staying within a specific, target range as much as humanly possible. Target ranges are generally in the same ballpark, but ultimately depend on age, daily routine, and stage of life. They are agreed upon with an endocrinologist because they are individualized and change over time. For example, my target range at the age of 23 is ~70-120 mg/dL (3.9-6.7 mmol/L), but as a child and teenager, it was ~80-180 mg/dL (4.4-10.0 mmol/L). Much broader with a larger buffer space for lows.

No matter the target range, it's the time spent within that range that matters most. How often do we fluctuate out of range? How drastically? And for how long? Temporarily spiking to 250 mg/dL (13.9 mmol/L) is very different than staying there for 5 hours straight. Frequency, amplitude, and time spent out of range contribute to hemoglobin A1C—the percent of red blood cells with glucose attached that indicates our average blood glucose over the past 2-3 months. In the 2017 "Standards of Medical Care in Diabetes," the American Diabetes Association (ADA) recommended teenagers shoot for an A1C ≤ 7.5% while adults shoot for an A1C ≤ 7.0%.[1] To translate these A1Cs to average blood sugars (estimated average glucose, eAG), we can use the formula:[2]

$$28.7 \times A1C - 46.7 = eAG$$

The recommendation of 7.5% equates to an average blood sugar of 169 mg/dL (9.4 mmol/L) while 7.0% would be around 154 mg/dL (8.6 mmol/L).

For reference, here is a list of A1C values and corresponding average blood sugars:

A1C %	Blood Sugar (mg/dL)	Blood Sugar (mmol/L)
4.0	68	3.8
4.5	82	4.6
5.0	97	5.4
5.5	111	6.2
6.0	126	7.0
6.5	140	7.8
7.0	154	8.5
7.5	169	9.4
8.0	183	10.2
8.5	197	11.0
9.0	212	11.7
9.5	226	12.6
10	240	13.3
11	269	15.0
12	298	16.6
13	326	18.1
14	355	19.7

While the A1C is currently the best indicator of overall control, it is not a perfect test and does not tell the entire story. There are people who reach A1C recommendations and have terrible control. They experience huge swings in their blood sugars (high variability) and many low blood sugars. Our aim is to have an A1C as low as possible while minimizing variability and low blood sugars.

Now that we know our *what*, let's explore some of our *wants*...why should tighter control be our aim?

The *Want*

We are too often given scary lectures about why we *should* work for tighter control. Although these little talks usually come from people with good intentions, they do not realize that fear is a poor motivator...especially at a young age when most people with T1D feel pretty invincible.

We don't train to escape bad situations, we train to create good ones. Runners do not run marathons because they are afraid of what may happen if they don't. Likewise, training for tighter control is something we *want* to do...not something we feel like we *should* do. The specific A1C targets we are encouraged to aim for are not arbitrary. Rather, they are guided by concrete results from the latest research that explores the health benefits we have to gain. Both right now and in the future. We work for positive changes in our management because of these daily and big-picture motivators.

Daily Motivators

"Most of anyone's life is a preoccupation with urgent inessentials. If we divide our affairs into what matters for a day or a season or the rest of our lives, it is the long-term fundamentals we give least time to, and put off till tomorrow's tomorrow. We are more concerned with the pressing than the important, and the essentials are easily crowded out by the mere day-to-day business of living."

- Nan Fairbrother, *The House in the Country*[3]

Because our management is constant, it can be easy to let it fade into the background and fall second to other, seemingly more urgent tasks. Yet when we reflect on all the ways in-range numbers help with what we might prioritize over management, it doesn't make much sense. In-range numbers reflect that the body and mind are able to function at their peaks, benefiting us physically, mentally, and even socially. This is achieved through a variety of interconnected health components, including:[4]

Energy

Glucose is the body's most important source of energy. It is used by every cell in the body. In fact, some cells, like those in the brain and nerves, *only* use glucose. The body was designed not to waste a single molecule. This means a standard amount allocated to the blood (~100 mg/dL (5.5 mmol/L)) and the rest allocated to tissues for immediate energy or stored energy in the form of glycogen.

However, when there isn't enough insulin on board (active insulin in circulation), tissues cannot properly take up glucose. Our bodies HAVE the energy, but aren't able to use it nor store it. As a result, we feel fatigued. During exercise when it is essential to have enough glycogen, performance can especially suffer.

One illustration is "carb-loading" in endurance sports such as marathon running. A higher volume of carbs is suggested to athletes because it allows muscles to store enough glycogen to get through long periods of exercise. However, it can be extremely challenging for athletes with T1D as there must be enough insulin on board to make use of the extra carbohydrates. Without insulin, carb-loading is completely useless and results in mega-high blood sugars. In-range numbers reflect that glucose is going to the right places and tissues have the energy they need now and later on.

Mental Clarity

Worrying about which direction our blood sugars are heading can be a major distraction when we are supposed to be focusing on other tasks. As we gain tighter control and lower variability, we face fewer "what if…?" questions and gain confidence that our numbers will be where we need them to be. This allows us to devote more attention to our lives outside of T1D.

Being out of range can also cloud our thinking and make us feel lightheaded or dizzy. Above or below range, the time it takes to complete tasks increases, reaction time is slower, and coordination is impaired. Being in range allows for sharp thinking, reactivity, and coordination; lending itself to scholastic and athletic performance. More importantly, in-range blood sugars increase safety in everyday activities like driving or using the stairs.

Hydration

As we learned (or will learn) in introductory chemistry, water follows solute. Glucose is solute and when extra glucose is in the blood, water is drained from tissues to compensate. This water then enters the blood and is filtered by the kidneys. The kidneys remove waste while conserving important molecules the body uses for energy and growth, such as glucose. However, when blood sugars reach what is called the renal threshold, (~180 mg/dL (10 mmol/L)),[5] the kidneys cannot properly conserve glucose. Instead, some glucose is removed in the urine. Again, water follows glucose and causes more frequent urination and consequently, dehydration.

Over half of the human body is water. Even a slight 1-2% loss of body water can impair physical and cognitive function.[6] Staying hydrated can supplement the boost in energy and focus we receive from in-range numbers. Not to mention, hydration is outwardly reflected in healthy, glowing skin that we rely on to protect us from harmful bacteria. With T1D, hydration also acts as a safeguard against the rapid acceleration of ketones.

Sleep Quality

Sleep disturbances are linked to higher chronic stress,[7] which can increase glucose-raising stress hormones such as cortisol. When blood sugars are stable and in range during sleep, we are less likely to be woken up. We avoid highs that lead to restroom trips and lows that lead to urgent, half-asleep sugary snacking. This improves our sleep quality by increasing the amount of restful sleep we get each night. In turn, our hormones are more balanced, making in-range numbers easier to achieve. Additionally, nothing can replace the supplemental boost in energy, focus, immunity, and outlook we get from a good night's sleep.

Satiety

When our bodies are running short on insulin, we feel more hungry...or worse, *hangry* (angry feelings that can accompany the sensation of hunger). In addition to delivering enough glucose to the body's cells, insulin helps signal to the brain that the body has the fuel it needs. This signal tells the brain to stop eating and gives us a feeling of fullness, or satiety. Without proper insulin, we are more likely to keep eating, even if we have all the fuel we need. And with lack of insulin and high blood sugars, eating more isn't exactly a good idea.

I find this to happen especially after meals when my insulin is timed too late. Even when I have eaten enough, if my blood sugar spikes and glucose isn't being delivered to my body's tissues, I am more tempted to snack or get seconds. Giving in usually leads to insulin stacking and an out-of-range number.

With enough insulin on board and the right timing, we feel full from the foods we eat. Blood sugars are less likely to spike after meals. And to the benefit of ourselves and those around us, we avoid feeling hangry.

Flexibility

Glucose is sticky. Dried juice on the floor? Sticky. Melted popsicle? Sticky. Excess glucose in the blood? Yes, also sticky. This stickiness can cause connective tissues like muscles, tendons, ligaments, and joints to move less readily over time. In-range numbers keep us flexible and protect us from suffering injuries. Additionally, muscle fibers that stretch a greater distance can produce stronger contractions, generating more force. More force = more powerful movements = increased athletic performance.

Immunity

Aside from connective tissues, excess glucose can cause trouble where germs (bad bacteria) congregate. Like our cells, germs prefer glucose and can use it to multiply. When the immune system cannot fight off the number of germs that accumulate, we end up with infections. Infections can manifest just about anywhere...especially in the nasal and throat passages, mouth, and skin. Since infections often increase insulin resistance, we can also end up with even higher blood sugars, providing more glucose for germs to multiply and making infections difficult to fight off.

By staying in range and doing our best to prevent infections, we spend less time away from school, work, and the activities we enjoy.

Outlook

Out-of-range numbers can be a huge source of mental strain. When they happen often, it's easy to become frustrated and lose confidence in our ability to manage T1D. Research has shown that out-of-range numbers are associated with feelings of depression, self-doubt, and lowered self-esteem.[8] Life gives us enough mental challenges already and T1D shouldn't add to them. In-range numbers take away these negative feelings to improve our relationships with ourselves (i.e., less negative self-talk) and others (i.e., more patience). In-range numbers can even act as a source of positivity...seeing that our hard work is paying off is something to be proud of.

Flexibility (again)

Being in range also gives us a chance to be metaphorically flexible. When we are unsure of where blood sugars are heading, we become more hesitant to say "yes" to spontaneous plans. Knowing what to expect from our blood sugars allows us to more readily adapt to in-the-moment opportunities. Kayaking, skydiving, impromptu excursions—with stable blood sugars we can do just about anything.

Big-Picture Motivators

There's a notable contrast between running recreationally and training for a race. Recreational running depends more on daily motivators without the bigger picture in mind. Runners have what they need to get out the door and finish a run, but not much beyond that.

When I run outside of training, I maintain an acceptable pace, but usually don't push myself to be faster. If the weather is bad, I'll find another workout. I may not finish my mileage, take the time to stretch properly, or do speed workouts—all the small, tedious things I know deep down I need to improve. I am satisfied by getting the job done and am less concerned with the quality of each run. Simply put: having big-picture motivators makes for a much better runner.

But even with big-picture motivators in mind, they can seem too distant to be real. At 16 weeks away from a marathon with the goal of a new personal record, there's so much between where I am and where I want to be. Hours and hours of time. Hundreds of miles. I sometimes ponder if small decisions really determine whether or not I reach that goal. Every rep of strengthening...the last half mile of a long run...refusing junk food...skipping out on late nights with friends for adequate sleep...is it truly making a difference?

The reality of reaching or not reaching that goal doesn't seem concrete until much closer to the actual race. Standing at the starting line, I am thankful for every single decision to follow through. Although I may not have fully realized it during training, those actions—no matter how small—prepared me for the moment that mattered most.

When I reflect on the possibility of ultimately not reaching a goal, I think back to the MCM. There are quite possibly small actions that might have made that 21-second difference. Perhaps if I could have taken medication to prevent the migraine. Or left the house five minutes earlier. Or have run mile 22 a little faster. Maybe I would have qualified for Boston. While I knew it wasn't the end of the world and I had more opportunities, questioning what I could have done differently was agonizing. And as agonizing as those questions were, it would have been devastating if that race was my only shot.

In this life with T1D, the race we're running *is* our only shot. Just like race day, we're eventually faced with the reality that we did everything we could do to achieve our goal, or we didn't. The last thing we want is to be asking "what if I had done x,y,z…?" Our big-picture motivator and #1 goal is a long, high-quality life without limitations. Preservation and even improvement of our current health. No matter how seemingly distant or abstract, this big-picture motivator is ever-present. And every small action we make accumulates toward reaching it.

Long-term studies have shown that working toward tighter control—even slight improvements—provides major protection. One of the most well-known studies is the Diabetes Control and Complications Trial (DCCT), which continued to become the Epidemiology of Diabetes Interventions and Complications (EDIC). The DCCT began in 1983 and compared people with T1D on conventional therapy (NPH and Regular insulin) to those on intensive therapy (basal/bolus with multiple daily injections (MDI) or pump therapy). After seven years, the two groups were compared. The group on conventional therapy had an average A1C of 9.2% while those on intensive therapy had an average A1C of 7.2%. More importantly, this improvement was associated with a 35-76% lower chance of developing complications and ~70% decrease in progression of already-existing complications.[9]

After the DCCT's completion, the same groups of people were followed up in the EDIC, which still continues as an ongoing, observational study. Guided by the results of the DCCT, treatment recommendations shifted to intensive therapy for all people with T1D and the differences in average A1C between the two groups narrowed. Both groups had an A1C ~8.0% after 17 years. However, results showed that those few years of tighter control for the group on MDI or pump therapy during the DCCT continued to help in protecting against complications.[10]

Note that this protection wasn't from reaching recommended A1Cs 100% of the time. It was from being *slightly* better. The fact that even small improvements over a few years continued to provide protective benefits two decades later shows us that control isn't an "all or none." In our care, every step counts in creating the highest quality of life for our future selves. In addition to daily motivators, tighter control lends itself to long-term health…specifically augmenting circulation, kidneys, nerves, pregnancy, and growth.

Circulation

Together, blood and blood vessels make up the circulatory system. Blood carries nutrients and oxygen (O_2) to the tissues, and then takes away waste products and carbon dioxide (CO_2). Arteries are the vessels that carry oxygenated blood away from the heart to the tissues. Veins are the vessels that retrieve deoxygenated blood from the tissues to bring back to the heart. This system gives organs continuous energy to perform their jobs.

To ensure every tissue in the body receives nutrients and O_2, vessels start off big near the heart (macrovessels), and then get smaller and smaller as they branch out (microvessels). In a healthy state, vessels are *adaptable*, swiftly adjusting to constantly changing conditions by expanding to increase blood flow to active tissues and constricting to shunt blood flow away from less-active tissues. Vessels are also *strong* and resistant to leakage and breaks. Finally, vessels are *clear* of inflammation, plaque buildup, and blood clots that could potentially cause high pressure or blockage.

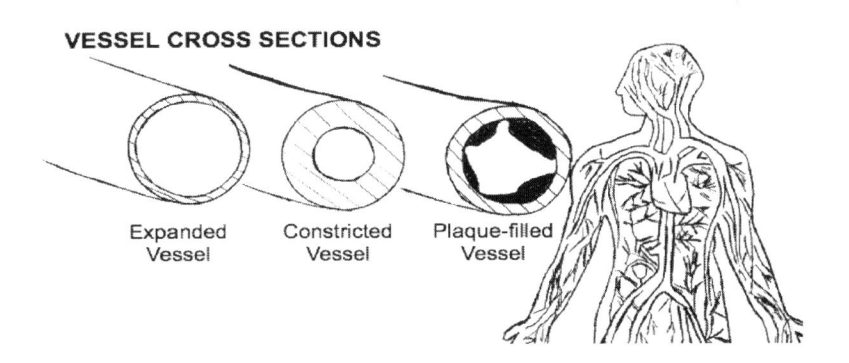

VESSEL CROSS SECTIONS

Expanded Vessel — Constricted Vessel — Plaque-filled Vessel

A rough sketch of the circulatory system. Healthy vessels expand and constrict as needed. Unhealthy vessels can become hardened and plaque-filled, increasing blood pressure and restricting blood flow.

In-range blood sugars preserve these functions as we age, helping to prevent:

- Retinopathy
  The retina is an area in the back of the eye that senses light. When vessels in the retina are damaged or partially blocked, new ones grow to supply enough blood flow. Damaged vessels are more prone to bursting and new vessels are fragile, both increasing the chance of blood leakage into retina tissue and impairment of normal vision.

- Heart attack
  With lack of blood flow to tissues, organs cannot function at their peak. With cessation of blood flow, organs may stop functioning altogether. While the heart pumps blood to the rest of the body, it also needs its own blood supply, which is provided by the coronary circulatory system. A heart attack results when there's a rupture or blockage in this system, and the heart does not receive the blood it needs to function.

- Stroke
  Similar to heart attacks, strokes occur from lack of blood flow due to blocked or ruptured vessels in the brain. Stroke outcomes depend on the severity and part of the brain that was affected.

- Slow healing
  Injuries need plenty of O_2 and nutrients from the blood to heal. The farther blood travels down a vessel, the greater the chance it will encounter damaged

areas that restrict blood flow. This is especially relevant in the extremities—arms, legs, hands, and feet. Since blood travels farthest to reach these areas, they can experience lack of blood flow and slow healing. Inconveniently, these areas are also where injuries like cuts, bruises, etc. tend to happen (especially if you're clumsy like me...).

Kidneys

After blood removes waste from tissues, it is filtered by the kidneys. The kidneys have millions of filtering units called nephrons that either recycle valuable molecules the body can use or permanently remove waste by excreting it into urine. Every day, our fist-sized kidneys filter about 180 liters of blood[11]—the amount of liquid in 180 large bottles of soda. A tall order for small organs!

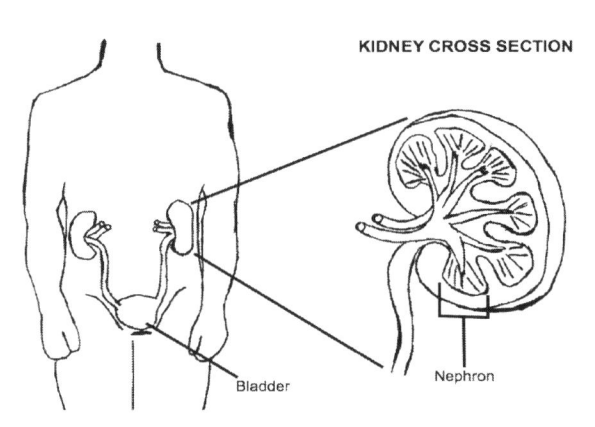

A simplified sketch of the kidneys, bladder, and kidney cross section. *Photo drawn with assistance from my lovely roommate, Liz Townsend.*

Excess glucose (and even other substances) in the blood can place additional stress on the kidneys as they work overtime to remove it and help maintain normal levels. When the kidneys are repeatedly stressed over time, they can start to lose their filtering ability, causing waste to accumulate in the blood. This can have a toxic effect on other organs—a process called nephropathy.

Nerves

The nervous system is a network of information pathways that allows the brain to communicate with the rest of the body. Nerves are designed for sensitivity, specificity, and most importantly, the fast relay of information.

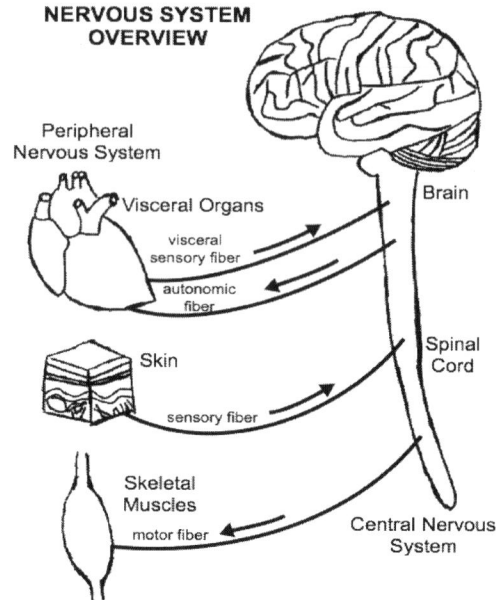

NERVOUS SYSTEM OVERVIEW

The central nervous system (brain and spinal cord) is in constant communication with organs in the peripheral nervous system.

Nerves have three major functions:

1) <u>Motor</u>: deals with movements in conscious thought—anything from simple tasks like hand clapping to complex skills like pole vaulting.
2) <u>Sensory</u>: deals with the five senses—sight, hearing, smell, touch, and taste. After the body picks up information from one of these senses, it is sent to the brain for interpretation (i.e., "Hot! Hand off stove." "Mmmm the smell of bacon...must be time to eat." "Ouch...I think I pulled a hamstring.").
3) <u>Autonomic</u>: deals with bodily functions outside of conscious thought such as heart rate, blood pressure, and digestion.

Nerve disease, or neuropathy, can be caused by a number of different conditions and affects motor, sensory, or autonomic function. In-range blood sugars preserve nerve tissue throughout the entire body, helping to prevent:

- Brain damage
  The brain is made up of large amounts of nervous tissue for memory storage and fast relay of information. Damage to this tissue can cause loss of memory and normal brain function. One such condition is Alzheimer's, which is characterized by fiber tangles within nerve cells and clusters of protein between nerve cells called plaques.

- Slow reaction time
  Although reaction time is mostly associated with quick starts in racing or hitting the buzzer first in a game show, it is even more essential for safety in everyday activities...especially ones like driving that involve frequent starting and stopping. When nerves in motor pathways are damaged, it takes longer for signals from the brain to reach the muscles. This can equate to slower reflexes and reaction times.

- Hypoglycemic unawareness
  When low blood sugars occur often over long periods of time, the body can lose the ability to sense them and send messages to the brain. Without these messages, the brain will not order the chemical signals that give us symptoms. No shaking, sweating, confusion, rapid heartbeat...in theory it sounds great! But in reality, it's dangerous. Those symptoms guard us so that we feel lows before we're *too* low. In-range numbers preserve these early warning signs.

- Inaccurate sensations
  When sensory nerves break down, the body can start feeling sensations when it shouldn't and NOT feeling sensations when it should. This is often called peripheral neuropathy as it primarily affects areas of the body farthest from the brain such as the feet and hands. Additional sensations from peripheral neuropathy include feelings of tingling and burning, while lack of sensation can cause numbness. Lack of sensation is especially dangerous as it could block *real* feelings of pain. Like symptoms of low blood sugar, feelings of pain serve as protection. By tending to pain, we treat injuries before they become worse. Instances of amputation are often because an injury wasn't taken care of right away and the site developed a serious infection that had to be kept from spreading.

- Delayed digestion
  The autonomic nervous system determines food's breakdown and speed of movement through the digestive tract. It is responsible for stimulating the involuntary movement of smooth muscles, changing blood flow, and secreting necessary chemicals and hormones. When nerves are not able to coordinate these actions in a timely manner, food takes longer to digest, a condition called gastroparesis. This can lead to bloating, gas, and even pain.

- Sexual dysfunction
  Sexual dysfunction is more related to T1D control in men compared to women,[12] and usually stems from autonomic neuropathy. This causes issues such as erectile dysfunction and retrograde ejaculation, both of which can lead to infertility.

- Orthostatic hypotension
  The body was designed to sense changes in position—sitting to standing to lying down, etc. Due to gravity, blood pressure needs to be higher when standing to help move blood from the feet back to the heart. When the autonomic nervous system doesn't respond quickly to increase blood pressure upon standing—also called orthostatic (upright) hypotension (low blood pressure)—it can cause symptoms of lightheadedness or dizziness.

Pregnancy

For women who want to have kids one day (even if that day is far, far away), in-range blood sugars are vital to healthy pregnancies. This includes normal fetal development, growth, and delivery. Glucose from the mother's blood can be transferred to the fetus, insulin cannot. When a mother's blood sugars run high, the developing fetus produces large amounts of insulin to compensate. Because the fetus receives an excess of nutrients from the mother's blood and insulin is an anabolic hormone that builds tissues, out-of-range blood sugars can lead to a larger-than-normal newborn (macrosomia). Tight control helps prevent macrosomia and protects the mother from developing complications.

Growth

Tight control helps children and teens reach their maximum growth potential, especially if they were diagnosed in early childhood. Adequate insulin and in-range blood sugars have been proven to increase the velocity of height growth and help achieve healthy body weight while lack of insulin and higher blood sugars have been shown to stall growth, leading to shorter stature and unhealthy body weight.[13]

A Holistic View

It's important to note these complications are not limited to only affecting people with T1D and a good number of people with T1D never experience any of these complications at all. Many things contribute to long-term health—early detection and a healthy lifestyle being two of them. In fact, many people say that having T1D makes them healthier than they would be otherwise, and it's logical to see why.

Because of T1D, we visit doctors regularly. If there are any problems in our health, they are likely to be caught and treated early. Not to mention, we receive a lot of health education. We know more than the average bear about living a healthy lifestyle and we practice our knowledge every single day. Finally, managing T1D puts our lives under a microscope—we see the effects of health decisions because they show in our blood sugars and insulin needs. Positive lifestyle choices boost our health relatively more compared to people without T1D because we gain protective benefits *and* benefits in day-to-day control. Therefore, we have extra motivation.

A healthy lifestyle includes staying away from harmful habits such as smoking and excessive drinking while practicing beneficial habits such as a balanced diet and regular physical activity. While both diet and physical activity should be customized to each individual's needs, there are certain recommendations that provide helpful guidance to all. Similar to the A1C, these recommendations are based on research of the short and long-term health benefits we have to gain.

Balanced Diet

> *"The food you eat can be either the safest and most powerful form of medicine or the slowest form of poison."*

-Ann Wigmore, founder of the Natural Health Institute

At the smallest, microscopic level, the foods we eat and our bodies are made up of the same substances. We eat food to grow and replenish. Our bodies are products of what we put into them over time. For better or worse, we are what we eat.

A healthy diet has the power to boost self-esteem, reduce stress and anxiety, create strong bones, regulate blood pressure, decrease vessel inflammation, boost immunity, enhance the body's antioxidant system, and protect against certain forms of cancer. Most importantly, food is the single largest determinant of body weight that we control. In the simplified "calories-in-calories-out" equation, SO many things contribute to "calories-out"...basal metabolic rate, thermogenesis, exercise...but only <u>one</u> thing contributes to "calories-in" and that's food. A balanced diet is the best route to a healthy body weight. All these benefits are ours for the taking with a diet consisting of the right number of high-quality Calories (kcals).

2,000 kcal/day is typically used as a reference amount on nutrition labels, but is only a rough estimate of what most people actually need. Each person's kcal intake should be completely individualized, depending on a number of different factors—age, sex, activity level, lean body mass, and health goals just to name a few. For the most customized healthy eating plan, it is best to consult with a registered dietitian. The Academy of Nutrition and Dietetics has online tools to find local registered dietitians, which can be found in Resources. The U.S. Department of Agriculture (USDA) also has great online tools that give more precise estimates of how many kcals a person needs for weight maintenance, loss, or gain.

There are three macronutrients that make up kcals—fat, carbs, and protein. Fat is the most energy dense at 9 kcal/gram while carbs and protein are both 4 kcal/gram. Fats usually make up ~25-35% of total kcals/day, carbs ~45-65%, and protein ~10-30%.[14] Again, these proportions depend on each individual and can be determined with the help of a registered dietitian.

It is important to note that **each macronutrient is essential.** Fats maintain normal hormone function, nerve health, and joint mobility. They also aid in the absorption of certain vitamins and increase satiety after meals. Carbs provide energy and fiber, which aids in blood sugar control and digestive health. Protein is used for synthesis and repair of muscles, bones, and skin. It makes up building blocks for enzymes and hormones. Importantly, each macronutrient provides vitamins the body does not produce on its own.

To maximize the benefits from each macronutrient, foods should be high-quality. Unfortunately when foods are processed, they are often stripped of the vitamins and minerals we need. Even when processed foods *do* have added vitamins and minerals, they are not in the combinations and amounts that only Mother Nature knows are best. The closer to nature, the better. The fewer unpronounceable ingredients, the better.

High-Quality Macronutrient Sources

Fats: Fish, nuts, seeds, olive oil, avocado

Carbs: Fruits, vegetables, dairy, whole grains, quinoa, beans

Proteins: Lean meats, seafood, dairy, nuts, seeds, beans, soy, eggs

Eating On-the-Go

In today's fast-paced world, efficiency is the name of the game. The faster, the better. The easier, the better. Unfortunately, this leads many people to reach for processed foods. They're convenient, yes. They're good, yes. But they're not good for you. These foods have low nutrient content and often leave us feeling hungry...that's actually part of the science behind processed foods to make us want more! With 1-2 minutes of planning, we can avoid the gimmicks and have the high-quality foods our bodies deserve. The snacks listed on the right are personal on-the-go favorites that provide proper nourishment. As an added bonus, these options also have a lower impact on blood sugars than most processed snack foods.

Quality On-the-Go Snacks

-whole fruits
-veggies + protein/fat (carrots, celery, snap peas, broccoli + ranch dressing, peanut butter, or hummus)
-whole-grain, low fat popcorn
-meat jerky
-nuts
-cheese sticks
-yogurt or cottage cheese
-tuna packets
-edamame, chickpeas (plain, dried, or roasted)
-boiled eggs
-whole wheat toast + protein/fat (cheese, peanut butter, or hummus)

pro tip: invest in good tupperware

The USDA's ChooseMyPlate.gov is a great tool for learning more about quality sources of macronutrients. It takes away some of the planning healthy eating requires by offering tips to reach recommended servings of essential food groups, recipes, and meal plans for all needs and budgets.

Regular Physical Activity

When it comes to physical activity, most people automatically pigeon-hole themselves into one of two categories: either they're active or they're not. But no matter the category we consider ourselves to be in, we are ALL active. Getting up to go to the bathroom...that's activity. Flipping the pages of this book...that's activity. Physical activity is a spectrum. And on that spectrum there are unhealthy levels of activity that are too low and unhealthy levels that are too high. Somewhere in the middle of these two extremes, there's a range of activity that provides maximum benefits—boosted self-esteem, reduced stress and anxiety, better sleep, healthy body weight, strong bones, regulated blood pressure, increased HDL cholesterol (the good kind), decreased LDL cholesterol (the bad kind), decreased vessel inflammation, enhanced antioxidant system, increased heart-pumping capacity, and greater muscle tone. And particularly notable to those of us with T1D, exercise improves insulin sensitivity by increasing glucose uptake into the muscles.

While a certain proportion of glucose uptake is influenced by factors beyond our control, the two factors we *do* control are insulin and physical activity. Aside from the liver, the muscles are a HUGE sink for storing glucose as glycogen. In fact, around 80% of the glucose we receive from food can be taken up by muscles.[15]

Insulin sensitivity increases acutely during activity when additional glucose-uptake receptors come to the surface of working muscles to remove glucose from the blood. These receptors are present during activity for instant energy and hours after activity to restore glycogen depots. When muscles grow from consistent exercise, our sink for glucose storage also grows and helps us maintain insulin sensitivity over time.

With improved insulin sensitivity, we can steer blood sugars more efficiently and decrease the severity of blood sugar swings. Since so much of our insulin regimen depends on our tracking abilities, having higher insulin:carb ratios and correction factors leave a little more wiggle-room for human error. Blood sugars are not as likely to spike as quickly or as high for someone who maintains insulin sensitivity. Accordingly, regular physical activity has been shown to improve control in youth with T1D.[16] Maintaining insulin sensitivity is also associated with cardiovascular protection and healthy blood pressure, triglyceride, and cholesterol levels.[17]

Currently, the U.S. Department of Health and Human Services (HHS) recommends 60+ minutes of physical activity a day for children and teens with most of those minutes at moderate or vigorous intensity. Activities should be muscle strengthening three days a week and bone strengthening three days a week. For adults over 18, the HHS recommends 150+ minutes a week of moderate activity or 75+ minutes a week of vigorous activity. Activities should be muscle strengthening at least two days a week.[18] Examples of these activities can be found online in the HHS's *Physical Activity Guidelines for Americans*.

To reap maximum benefits and ensure consistent levels of insulin sensitivity, spreading activity out over the course of the week is more effective than packing all activity into one day. Finally, if you are not currently meeting recommendations, hope is not lost. ALL activity matters. Some is better than none and even small choices add up. Do what you *can* do and what you *like* to do. Tips for increasing physical activity can be found at USDA's ChooseMyPlate.gov as well as other professional health organizations listed in Resources.

Make It Personal

Motivation is highly personal and changes over time. We can be driven by one motivator, or a combination of motivators all at once. We find our strongest motivation by reflecting on our values...the type of person we strive to be, what we hope to achieve, and the impact we hope to have. How do our daily and big-picture motivators help to get us there?

Below is a section for self-reflection. The answers provided are there to help brainstorm!

Reflections

How would my life benefit from improved _____?

Energy
An enthusiastic audition for a role in the school play, picking up a new workout routine after school

_____

_____

Focus
Scoring higher on calculus tests, producing top-notch work at my new job, beating Dad in a game of chess

_____
_____

Hydration
Better football practices and earning a starting position

_____
_____

Sleep Quality
Feeling relaxed and refreshed, not falling asleep in class

_____
_____

Flexibility
Lower chance of injury, achieving a new 1-rep max on the bench press

_____
_____

Satiety
Fewer impulsive, low-quality snack foods, being more comfortable at work during the long stretch between breakfast and lunch

_____
_____

Immunity
Fewer missed days of work, less money spent on avoidable doctor's visits

_____
_____

Outlook/Metaphorical Flexibility
Greater resilience when things inevitably go wrong, making new friends at a new school, saying "yes" more often to spontaneous plans

_____

_____

Long-term Protection
Meeting my grandchildren (or great grandchildren), winning the Boston Marathon in the Master Women's category, earning a 75-year medal from the Joslin Diabetes Center

_____

_____

Once we have a clear vision of how tighter control changes our lives for the better, we're ready to equip ourselves with the knowledge to do the job…continuously learning how to best tackle the task at hand.

PART II

LEARNING (AND RELEARNING) ABOUT THE TASK AT HAND

The year was 490 B.C. when the Persian army arrived in Marathon, Greece ready to fight. After multiple successful attacks, they were poised to win the final battle that would let them conquer the Greeks once and for all. The Greek army was heavily outnumbered and not nearly as prepared, but had no other choice—they would defend their freedom and pride at all costs.

Against all odds, the Greek army fought the battle of a lifetime. They defeated the Persians and saved their entire country! Eager to share the news of their victory, they sent one of their best athletes, Philippides, to run 25 miles from Marathon to Greece's capital in Athens. No one gave it a second thought. What was 25 miles after defeating the Persian army?

As fast as he could, Philippides made his way to Athens. Upon arrival, he proclaimed, "Rejoice, we conquer!" Then he dropped dead. Running 25 miles is clearly not something the human body was designed to do on a whim.

Nevertheless, inspired by the legend of Philippides, the marathon became an Olympic event and is now a popular bucket list item for crazy people like myself. At a slightly longer length of 26.2 miles, millions of people have gone the distance. Most of them without keeling over.

How is this possible when not even one of ancient Greece's best athletes could run a marathon? Well, humans did not evolve into better athletes. What *did* evolve was our understanding of physiology and training techniques. Over the years, the human mind has learned to overcome the body's limitations. Guided by research and a rich history of trial and error, we now know how to prepare the body for a nonstop 26.2-mile run.

At a glance, this includes: the amount of time needed to train (~16-20 weeks); mileage build up (usually increasing long runs by a mile each week until reaching 18-22 miles, and then tapering off three weeks prior to a race); eating in the days and hours before a race (carb-loading to build up glycogen stores), during a race (fast-acting glucose every 30-45 minutes to help conserve glycogen stores), and after a race (meal with ~2:1 ratio of carbs to protein within 45 minutes of finishing); cross-training methods (strengthening and low-impact exercises like swimming, yoga, or cycling); and avoiding injuries (using foam rollers, support wraps, and ALWAYS warming up before and stretching after runs). Like any sporting event, it's specific training for a specific task.

As time goes on, the body of knowledge and resources for running marathons will continue to grow and runners will be able to train more efficiently. From the time I started writing this book in May 2015 to the time I am revising this paragraph in December 2017, a new world marathon record was set at 2:00:25 by Eliud Kipchoge.[1] This is a pace of 4:36 min/mile and nearly an entire hour faster than the 1908 record of ~2:55:00.[2] Crazy.

Despite this impressive pace, 2:00:25 was actually a relative disappointment. This new record is part of Nike's Breaking2 project—a collaboration of the best athletes and scientists in the world to achieve a sub 2-hour marathon. The quest to achieve a sub 2 started when sports physiologist,

Michael Joyner, created a model of marathon performance that predicted the time of a physiologically-ideal marathon runner in a perfect setting to be 1:57:58.[3] To make this time a reality, Breaking2 engages some of the world's most skilled runners—Olympic Marathon champion, Eliud Kipchoge, half marathon world record holder, Zersenay Tadese, and up-and-comer, Lelisa Desisa—who were chosen based on their high levels of maximal oxygen consumption and lactate threshold as well as their resilient mentalities.

Every detail of their training is tightly monitored. This ranges from physiological markers like muscle glycogen and hydration to clothing and shoes. Finally, these runners are put to the test on the highly-controlled Formula One track. Its location in Monza, Italy allows for a flat course with ideal altitude, humidity, and temperature for springtime racing. While attempting a sub 2, runners are flanked by a rotating group of pacers to create an ideal drafting pattern. Meanwhile, a car with an enormous digital clock drives ahead of the pack for pacing.[4] With optimization of every small detail, there will undoubtedly be a runner who drops the half second required for a sub 2-hour marathon.

Equally if not more outstanding is the progression of knowledge in understanding and treating T1D. We haven't even hit the 100-year anniversary of insulin therapy. Exactly 100 years ago, an optimistic prognosis for someone with T1D was living a few low-quality years after diagnosis. Some patients were prescribed strange diets consisting mostly of animal products (i.e., meats, milk, and "blood pudding") as some physicians correctly suspected that carbs contributed to sugar in the urine. A contradicting belief was that people with T1D needed higher amounts of sugar in their diets because they lost so much in their urine. Additional treatments included opium, arsenic, alcohol, and purgatives.[5]

Since those times, we have progressively gained a better understanding of T1D. And beyond an understanding, we have found effective therapies for treatment. Combined with advanced technology, this has revolutionized the way we live with T1D.

We owe the quantity and quality of life we have today to constant discovery. What may seem like common knowledge now is the result of countless lives' work to find:

Which organs control glucose in the blood?
What is the role of the pancreas in T1D?
How does insulin work? How can it be replaced in someone who doesn't make any themselves?
How does injected insulin best mimic the pattern of insulin secreted by beta cells?
How can insulin delivery be more precise? More convenient?
What type of treatment regimens give the best outcomes?

Answers to questions like these built the foundation for T1D treatments, both in the past and today. Small actions in our management are specifically designed from this knowledge to mimic the body's natural physiology. Like running marathons, it's specific training for a specific task. The more we learn about the task we are training for and the techniques we can use to accomplish that task, the more informed we are in our management decisions. Every lesson is a tool and knowing the importance of each action in our care gives us motivation to follow through.

Our Task

The body was designed to have a fixed range of glucose in the bloodstream at all times (~100 mg/dL ± 20 mg/dL (~5.6 ± 1.1 mmol/L)) to ensure tissues have the energy they need without being stressed by excess glucose. This range is achieved through a constant balance of hormones that increase or decrease blood sugars as needed. While many hormones increase blood sugars, the hormone most associated with this function is glucagon. And as we are very familiar with, the main hormone to decrease blood sugars is insulin.

To determine which hormone is needed and how much, a small fraction of cells in the pancreas called the islets of Langerhans—specifically alpha and beta cells—act as a sensor. When more glucose is

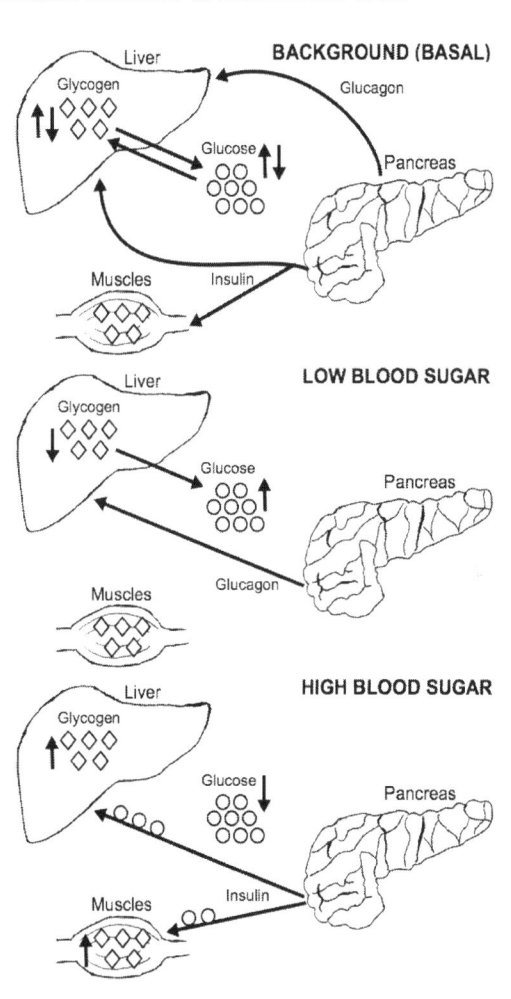

Our task in a nutshell. Insulin and glucagon are released throughout the day to adapt to the body's changing needs. More glucagon is released in response to low blood sugars while more insulin is released in response to high blood sugars.

needed in the blood, alpha cells release glucagon to act on the liver. Along with the muscles, the liver is a major source of glycogen. In response to glucagon, the liver breaks down glycogen and releases it as glucose into the bloodstream. In fact, the liver was designed to release small bits of glucose throughout the entire day. This is how the body prevents low blood sugars between meals...particularly at night when humans spend half a day without food.

When there is an excess of glucose in the blood, beta cells release insulin. Insulin allows tissues to take in glucose for energy and storage—especially the liver and muscles due to their capacity to store large amounts of glycogen. Insulin is released both after meals in bulk (bolus) and throughout the day in small amounts (basal) to counteract the liver's constant glucose release.

When beta cells are destroyed thanks to our overzealous autoimmunity, we are left with the task of regulating blood sugars on our own. To act as a sensor, we use self-monitored blood glucose (SMBG) testing. To increase blood sugars, we use carbs. To decrease blood sugars, we use insulin. Simple enough, right?

You already know the answer—of course not! That's because no one is smart enough and no tools are sophisticated enough to recreate the body's intricate balance. Even though we've come a long way in treating T1D, we work with a lot of limitations that can make our task exceedingly difficult.

Our first limitation is sensing changes in blood sugars. Alpha and beta cells do this continuously. All 86,400 seconds of the day. By using SMBG testing, we only get snapshots of a continuous story. Since we don't spend every second of every day testing, we're left with large gaps of time when we don't know what our blood sugars are doing.

A second limitation is that injected insulin is slow compared to the insulin released by beta cells. After meals, bolus insulin from beta cells starts working in less than ten minutes and finishes its job within an hour whereas commonly used rapid-acting injected insulin starts working in about 15 minutes and finish in about 3-5 hours.[6]

A third limitation is that injected insulin is inflexible. Normally, insulin levels decrease when blood sugars start falling (i.e., during exercise) and increase when they start rising (i.e., after meals). But injected insulin is much less fun and spontaneous than we are. The amount of insulin we take stays on board until it's finished working no matter what. Combined with poor sensing ability, the inflexible nature of our insulin means we are more likely to experience fluctuations in blood sugars, especially from food, physical activity, and changes in insulin sensitivity.

Promisingly, methods to overcome these limitations continue to advance, making it more feasible for us to tackle the challenges of our task and achieve tighter control.

Acting as a Sensor

Just like alpha and beta cells, before we do anything to steer blood sugars in another direction, we have to answer two important questions: Where is our blood sugar at right now? Where is it going?

Unlike alpha and beta cells, we unfortunately don't know the answers automatically. Symptoms often don't come until we're already out of range and even then, they can be confusing. Highs can feel like lows, lows like highs, and normal feelings of nervousness or fatigue can make us feel out of range when we're not. It doesn't matter if we've had T1D for 20 days or 20 years—we can never assume blood sugars. The only way to know is by using our data.

Without a continuous glucose monitor (CGM), the ADA recommends SMBG testing around 6-10 times a day: before meals for accurate insulin calculations and before bed to prevent nighttime lows. They also recommend testing prior to exercise, when we suspect a low blood sugar, after treating a low, and before activities that necessitate concentration for safety, like driving (especially for long periods of time).[8] Simply put, we need to know blood sugars before we do anything that may change them.

Hasty treatment decisions not based on blood sugar readings are dangerous and are more likely to lead to out-of-range numbers. Sound decisions are based on current blood sugar readings and are taken from a clean site using fresh supplies. After all, blood samples are tiny. Even just a little bit of residual sugar on the skin makes a huge difference.

My sister, Brooke, and I learned this lesson the hard way as kids when we tested her blood sugar for fun. She had just eaten a piece of fruit and we wanted to see what her after-meal blood sugar was like. We got a reading of 300 mg/dL (16.7 mmol/L) and immediately told my mom who was probably on the verge of a heart attack. Before rushing Brooke to the emergency room, we wiped her hand with an alcohol swab, changed the lancet, and tried again. 110 mg/dL (6.1mmol/L). A two-fold difference...all because of a little fruit residue on the fingers. And on that note, we shouldn't hesitate to test again when we have doubts about a reading.

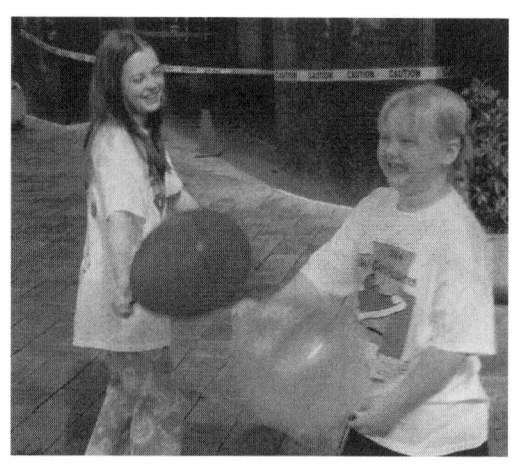

Brooke (right) and me (left) at the JDRF OneWalk in Washington, D.C. eight months after I was diagnosed.

After we're sure of our number, we come to the second question: where is it going? Having an idea of blood sugar and insulin context can make a huge difference in treatment decisions. For example, going on a walk at a steady 120 mg/dL (6.7 mmol/L) with no active insulin is a lot different than going on a walk at 120 mg/dL (6.7 mmol/L) after dropping 60 mg/dL (3.3 mmol/L) in 30 minutes with 2 units of insulin on board.

Context of a reading could determine how far we walk, the intensity, if we eat anything beforehand...it could mean the difference between being safe or being stranded with a low blood sugar. Knowing context also helps us avoid "insulin stacking"—not giving a previous bolus the time it needs to work, and then reacting to an out-of-range number by taking more insulin unnecessarily.

Just like blood sugar readings, we can never make assumptions about context. We can only work with the facts. This includes: additional SMBG readings, CGM readings, and active insulin.

The more SMBG readings we have, the clearer the picture we create. It's like a flipbook. With four separate images during a marathon, we may be able to tell that a runner was at the starting line, ran, crossed the finish line, and got a medal. But who's to say this runner didn't start the race, jump in a taxi, eat three doughnuts, and then run just the last quarter mile? (There was once a runner in the Boston Marathon who did something similar). With more pictures in time, we would be more likely to create the entire story. Likewise, when we test more often and vary the times of our testing, we connect the dots to create a better picture of what our blood sugars are doing throughout the day. Studies have even shown that testing more often is associated with better outcomes in glycemic control and lower A1Cs.[9]

Glucose (mg/dL)

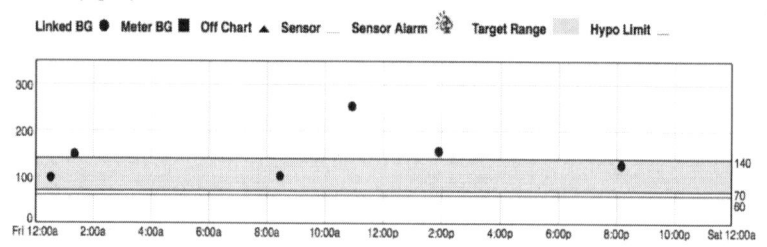

The extra, out-of-range SMBG reading after breakfast suggests that insulin was not timed properly. Image from Medtronic CareLink software.

CGM data also gives us an idea of our numbers and context. Readings are taken every 1-5 minutes (depending on the device) from glucose in the interstitial fluid that surrounds the cells. It is not taken from blood glucose. Therefore, there can be a lag between blood sugars and CGM readings. Additionally, most CGM devices depend on SMBG testing to stay accurate.[‡] Blood sugar readings have to be entered into a CGM system throughout the day for calibrations. This ensures the interstitial fluid properly reflects blood sugars. With that said, CGM readings offer incredibly useful insight to context and can help us see what is happening in the time between blood sugar checks.

Glucose (mg/dL)

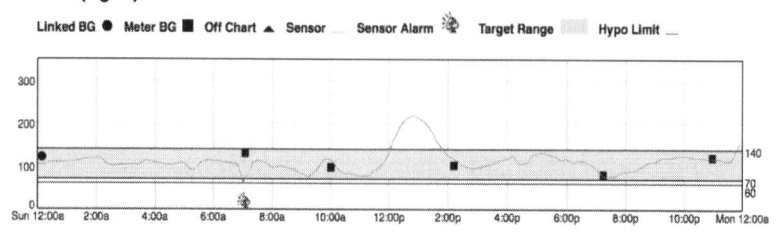

Without the CGM tracing, we would not be able to see the post-lunch spike since all SMBG readings are in range. Image from Medtronic CareLink software.

[‡] There are certain CGM devices recently approved by the FDA that do not require SMBG testing for calibrations such as Abbott's FreeStyle Libre or Dexcom's G6.

Personally, using a CGM helped me trust that bolusing in advance and using a "super bolus" when I was sedentary helped decrease my blood sugar spikes after meals without causing lows (more on super bolusing to come in a few pages). It has also provided earlier warnings of low blood sugars, helping to prevent them.

Active insulin (also called "insulin on board") is insulin that is still working from a previous bolus dose. Active insulin depends on the time a bolus was taken, how many units were given, and how long the insulin is expected to work. An insulin pump keeps track of this information automatically. Most pumps even take active insulin into consideration when calculating new bolus doses. Technology such as smartphone apps and gadgets for insulin pens have also made it a lot easier to track active insulin. Examples are listed in Resources.

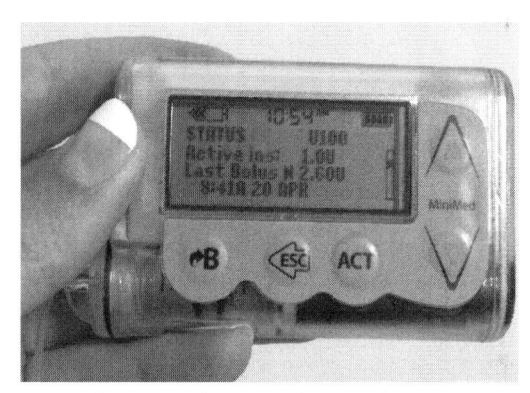

Medtronic insulin pump display of estimated insulin on board 2 hours after a breakfast bolus.

Sans technology, we can roughly estimate active insulin by multiplying the dose amount by (time passed/time of insulin action).[10] For example, after taking an 8-unit bolus of rapid-acting insulin that takes ~4 hours to finish working, there would be ~2 units on board after 3 hours (8 units x ¾ = 2 units).

Minimizing Fluctuations

Inevitably, we do at least three things that regularly change our blood sugars—take insulin, eat, and move around. Minimizing fluctuations from these necessary activities is possible with proactive planning and strategic choices. Often, the biggest challenge is balancing insulin needs with one or both of the other activities. Since our insulin is inflexible, many techniques for minimizing fluctuations are meant to accommodate insulin action—both in timing and amount. Here are a few tools that I have found particularly helpful:

After Eating

When it comes to balancing insulin with food, the most basic consideration is grams of carbs. The amount of carbs reflects how much blood sugars are expected to rise from a meal and therefore, gives us an idea of the insulin needed to compensate. The insulin:carb component of our bolus calculation (not counting correction factor) is the expected amount to put us back at our premeal blood sugars 3-5 hours later. Any time prior to 3 hours and blood sugars have likely not come down fully from the last bolus. For this reason, it's also helpful to spread out meals rather than constantly snacking and bolusing throughout the day.

So what's going on in those 3-5 hours after we eat? Our blood sugars will go up with carbs and come down with insulin, but this peak can happen in a number

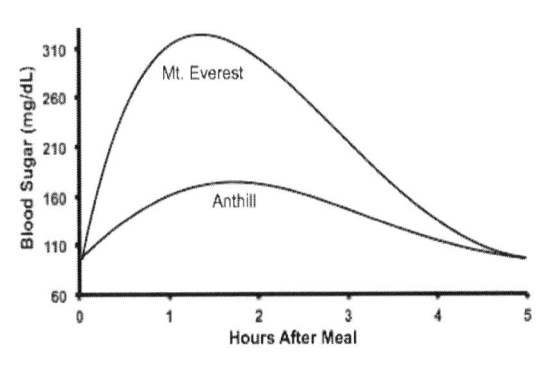

Focusing on insulin timing and food composition can lower post-meal spikes.

of ways. Will it resemble an anthill, or Mt. Everest? The better carb digestion matches insulin action, the smaller our peak. Currently, the ADA recommends that teens with T1D aim for blood sugars below 200 mg/dL (11 mmol/L) after meals while adults stay under 180 mg/dL (10 mmol/L).[11, 12]

This can present a challenge. As we mentioned before, insulin from beta cells starts working almost immediately while injected insulin takes substantially longer. In addition, beta cells secrete a less-talked-about hormone, amylin, that slows down digestion. Since we don't have the luxury of beta cells, we work with slower insulin *and* we don't have amylin. Together, this means carbs typically absorb faster than insulin begins working.

The first line of defense for matching carb digestion and insulin action is bolusing before meals. It has even been shown that bolusing with rapid-acting insulin 20 minutes prior to eating leads to smaller spikes and significantly better blood sugars 1 and 2 hours after a meal compared with bolusing right before a meal or 20 minutes after.[13]

With that said, boluses still depend on context. The official recommendation from the ADA is "match prandial (mealtime) insulin to carbohydrate intake, premeal blood glucose, and anticipated physical activity."[14] For example, if I am not able to move around much after a meal (i.e., at work) or am out-of-range, bolusing in advance works really well. But right before a workout, I know I will be fine with a small bolus right at mealtime...or no bolus at all depending on the amount of carbs and nature of the exercise. And if we're unsure of the time we'll be eating (i.e., at restaurants), bolusing in advance can be dangerous.

It can also be difficult to take a premeal bolus when we don't know what we'll be eating (i.e., in a school cafeteria). When this is the case, I find that taking a conservative bolus—even if it ends up not covering the entire amount of carbs—helps with post-meal blood sugars. For example, if I know that I'll have at least 15 carbs, I'll take a bolus early for that amount. Then if I actually have 30 carbs, I take another bolus for 15 carbs just before the meal. In case a meal isn't what we expected it to be, it's a good idea to keep a snack with carbs on hand such as a granola bar and always, fast-acting glucose.

The second line of defense is considering the type of carbs we're eating. 20 carbs of carrots would require the same amount of insulin as 20 carbs of glucose tabs. But in the 3-5 hours it takes to come back to baseline, would blood sugar peaks look the same if insulin were taken at the same time? No.

Not all carbs are created equal. Carbs digest at different rates due to a food's composition. Quickly-digested carbs cause faster glucose release into the bloodstream and

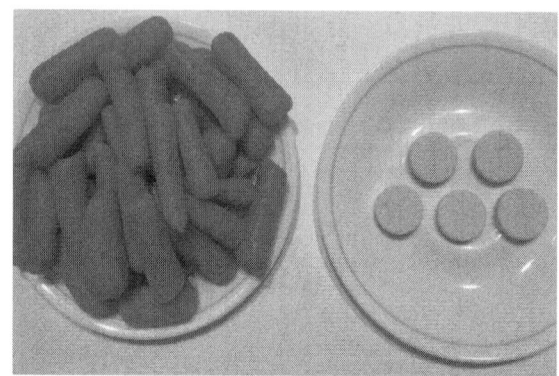

20 carbs of carrots versus 20 carbs of glucose tabs...that's A LOT of carrots.

create a more pronounced peak while slowly-digested carbs result in slower glucose release and a more subtle peak. Not to mention, carbs that digest slower help us feel fuller longer and their gradual glucose release allows for sustained energy.

The time it takes for different foods to increase blood sugar levels is described by the Glycemic Index (GI). The GI is a scale from 0-100 that corresponds to the percent of carbs released into the bloodstream as glucose within 2 hours of eating. The closer to 0, the slower the glucose release. The closer to 100, the faster the glucose release. Glucose itself is set at 100 as the reference point because it is already in the form of sugar the body needs. It takes little digestion time and increases blood sugars most rapidly.

Other foods fall into three categories based on their timing of glucose release compared to that of pure glucose: high (70-100), moderate (56-69) and low (0-55). Examples of foods in each category include:[15]

High GI	**Moderate GI**	**Low GI**
White bread	Pineapple	Carrots
Corn flakes	Sweet potato	Apples
Rice cakes	Popcorn	Chickpeas
Russet potatoes	Steel cut oats	Kidney beans
Watermelon	Quinoa	Grapefruit
Pretzels	Brown rice	Green veggies
Gatorade	Sweet corn	Premium ice cream *note that "low GI" does not equate to "healthy"

Because only a few institutions worldwide have the capacity to do the specialized testing GI scoring requires, most foods are not labeled with their GI values. However, we can get an idea of a food's GI value by looking at its:

- Fiber, protein, and fat
  Fiber, protein, and fat take longer to digest, therefore lowering a food's GI value.

- Acidity
  Foods that contain acidic ingredients such as vinegar or lemon juice will be lower on the GI than comparable, less-acidic foods.

- Ripeness
  Fruits and veggies that are less ripe tend to be lower on the GI while ripe fruits and veggies tend to be higher.

- Preparation
  Cooked foods tend to be higher on the GI. For example, raw carrots have a GI value of 35 while boiled carrots have a GI value of 49.[16] Processed foods also tend to be higher on the GI as they have been stripped of the fiber and nutrients that slow digestion.

GI value is an average of *all* the foods present in a meal. For example, we can lower the GI value of a plain bagel (69)[17] by adding cream cheese because it contains protein and fat.

Overall impact on blood sugars depends on both number of carbs and GI value. This is described by the Glycemic Load (GL):[18]

$$GL = (\# \text{ of carbs} \times GI \text{ value})/100$$

In a nutshell: fewer carbs and foods lower on the GI minimize a meal's impact on blood sugars. We can use this information to decrease post-meal spikes in a few ways...

First, we can be sure that most meals contain items lower on the GI. When we don't have the chance to take insulin in advance, eating items lower on the GI first can slow digestion and give insulin the head start it needs. And in the event that we are not positive about a meal's carb count, a more gradual rise in blood sugars gives us additional time to decide if we'll need more insulin before we go *too* high.

A number of different studies around the world have found that diets containing a good amount of low GI foods help improve blood sugar control and lower the risk of developing complications.[19] Does this mean we should only eat low GI foods? No! All foods have their time and place. Many healthy foods have high or moderate GI values. With low blood sugars and certain endurance sports, we *need* fast-acting carbs. For us, food is a tool. The more we know about the amount and type we eat, the better we can coordinate food and insulin to achieve in-range numbers.

Second, if we know a meal is higher on the GI, we can lower its impact by:

1) giving insulin further in advance,
2) eating a smaller portion, or
3) moving more after eating to increase insulin sensitivity (even something as small as walking for ten minutes).

If using an insulin pump, we can also consider using a super bolus to minimize post-meal spikes. This is when a reduced, temporary basal is set after a meal and that insulin is added onto the bolus dose. For example, with a basal of 0.5 units/hour, a 2-hour temporary basal at 20% of normal (0.1 units/hour) would mean taking an additional 0.8 units with a bolus dose. This increased insulin up front can decrease post-meal spikes while avoiding lows later on.[20] More information on super boluses can be found in *Pumping Insulin* by John Walsh and Ruth Roberts, listed in Resources. Before adjusting strategies for dosing insulin, it is always best to consult with an endocrinologist or certified diabetes educator (CDE).

We know the foods we like to eat and we eat them often. Taking the time to learn how to stay in range after eating our favorite foods is a high-yield investment that pays off over and over. If we minimize post-meal spikes, theoretically eat three times a day, and our insulin takes ~4 hours to work, that equates to 12 hours of better control. Half the day. Half our A1Cs.

Today, information about carb counts, portion sizes, and GI values are easily accessible. There are sites, apps, and books devoted to nutritional content for specific foods and restaurant items. Some examples can be found in Resources.

During and After Physical Activity

With functional beta cells, insulin levels fall during exercise while stress hormones rise to stimulate glucose release from the liver. This combination keeps blood sugars stable while providing muscles additional glucose for increased work.

Because our insulin levels don't fall naturally, finding the right strategies for exercising with T1D is the ultimate balancing act. We need carbs to fuel our activities. We need insulin to burn fuel properly and prevent ketones, especially during exercise when we're more likely to become dehydrated. Too many carbs and we risk high blood sugars, dehydration, and impaired performance. Too much insulin and we risk going low, decreasing our coordination and probably stopping our activity altogether.

Finding the right combination of carbs and insulin for a particular type of activity depends on a number of different factors, including:

- Intensity
  Typically, activities that are higher in intensity have a greater impact on insulin sensitivity. Aerobic activities like walking or dancing tend to decrease glucose during the activity itself while some high-intensity activities can cause blood sugars to rise before falling later on. The latter happens most often during activities that cause a temporary adrenaline rush (a part of the "fight or flight" acute stress response). Since adrenaline is a stress hormone, it acts on the liver to cause glucose release into the bloodstream. Examples of these activities include weightlifting, sprinting, and judged sports like gymnastics or figure skating (during skating competitions, I almost always experienced high blood sugars before my performance, and then a "crash" a few hours later).

- Duration
  The longer an activity is performed, the greater potential it has to decrease blood sugars.

- Training
  As the body becomes more adapted to an activity, it increases efficiency and less energy is required to perform the same task. Therefore, familiar activities decrease blood sugars less than new activities performed at a similar intensity and duration.

- Timing

    The body's reaction to an activity is affected by the time of day it is performed. Many people with T1D find their blood sugars are most stable while exercising in the morning when levels of circulating insulin are relatively low (this definitely held true during marathon training. Luckily, races are typically held in the morning!). Timing of the last bolus is a huge contributor to circulating insulin levels. Reducing bolus insulin is typically used for activities performed less than 90 minutes after a bolus dose while reducing basal insulin or supplementing with carbs is typically used for activities with no bolus adjustment.[21] When reducing bolus insulin, I found it helpful to take a certain % of my recommended dose depending on the activity. For example, I take 10-15% of my recommended bolus dose before long runs and 50% of my recommended bolus dose before teaching Pilates.

Sometimes people also experience delayed-onset hypoglycemia. These lows happen after an activity—sometimes hours later—and come from the body's need to replace lost glycogen stores. One way to combat this issue is by proper post-exercise nutrition.

After exercise, there is a critical window of time when the body restores glycogen most rapidly. The American College of Sports Medicine recommends refueling within 30 minutes after activity with the appropriate amount of carbs (~1-1.5 gram/kilogram of body weight)[22] and protein (~2:1 ratio of carbs to protein for moderate exercise and a ratio ~3:1 for high intensity).[23] To meet this recommendation, I try to time workouts before meals to ensure proper refueling without taking in unnecessary calories.

Of course, post-exercise nutrition depends entirely on the intensity and duration of the activity. The type of workout that elicits refueling usually involves sweating and elevated heart rate for long periods of time. For example, refueling may not be needed after a 30-minute yoga class, but would probably be necessary after a fast-paced, 90-minute soccer game.

Certain activities may not necessitate changes in carbs or insulin at all. A bout of resistance training or a lunchtime walk, for example. Or maybe blood sugars start off higher and exercise brings them back in range. It all depends on the individual, the activity, and the conditions of the day. This is what makes exercise so tricky.

Learning more about what happens physiologically while the body performs specific activities can offer useful insight in finding combinations of carbs, insulin, and timing that work best. Dr. Sheri Colberg is a sports physiologist with T1D who studies a variety of physical activities from triathlons to basketball to horseback riding and everything in between. She goes more in depth about the physiology and strategies for specific activities in *Diabetic Athlete's Handbook: Your Guide to Peak Performance*. Her work helped me form a framework for balancing T1D with marathon running, skating, dancing, and teaching fitness classes.

Because strategies for exercise are individualized, much of control during physical activity hinges on our ability to learn from our own experiences. We'll talk more about experienced-based learning in Part III.

When we don't know what exactly an activity will throw our way, it's a good idea to stay prepared by having double the amount of fast-acting glucose we think we may need. And if we are uncertain about intensity and duration, performing an activity with low levels of circulating insulin can be a safeguard against lows.

Changes in Insulin Sensitivity

Beyond our own actions, blood sugars can fluctuate due to changes in insulin sensitivity. Because insulin sensitivity depends on a number of transient factors, the same amount of insulin can cause blood sugars to drop more (increased sensitivity) or less (decreased sensitivity) than normal. Determinants of insulin sensitivity affect glucose uptake, glucose release, or both.

Both people with and without T1D experience changes in insulin sensitivity. With properly functioning alpha and beta cells, the body effortlessly adapts glucagon and insulin levels to maintain stable blood sugars. But without those capabilities, changes in insulin sensitivity can make for unpleasant blood sugar swings, even when we do everything right. This is because basal and bolus doses are based on assumed levels of sensitivity. And that level of sensitivity is based on a typical day under normal conditions.

A typical day under normal conditions…is real life the same day over and over? No. We get sick. We travel. We grow. We change jobs. We go on hikes. All of these changes in routine are normal, yet pretty much all of them can change insulin sensitivity.

So what do we do? Many determinants of insulin sensitivity are beyond our immediate control. And we don't know how certain determinants will affect us. Even within the same person, response to determinants of insulin sensitivity may change over time.

Strategizing for changes in insulin sensitivity always depends on the unique individual and situation. Like physical activity, it hinges on learning from personal experience. The best thing we can do is go over results regularly and use our trends as clues.

Determinants of Insulin Sensitivity, Typical Patterns[24]	
Physical Activity -more = ↑ sensitivity -less = ↓ sensitivity	**Stress Levels** -less = ↑ sensitivity -more = ↓ sensitivity
Environment -extreme temperatures, high humidity, and high altitude can lead to ↑ OR ↓ sensitivity depending the body's use of glucose and stress factors *moral of the story: keep an eye on trends to catch this early on	**Illness/Infection** -infections often = ↓ sensitivity *note: stomach illness can decrease blood sugars if food does not get the proper chance to absorb
Ingested Non-Carbs -medications (varies) -caffeine = ↓ sensitivity -protein in absence of carbs/bolus = ↓ sensitivity	**Body Composition** -increased lean mass = ↑ sensitivity -increased fat mass = ↓ sensitivity
Alcohol -typically increases blood sugars initially due to carbs found in alcoholic beverages with a drop later on as the liver cleanses alcohol from the bloodstream and does not release normal amounts of glucose	**Hormone Levels** -varies depending on: -time of day (i.e., circadian rhythm) -season -aging (higher levels of stress hormones in teenage years can cause ↓ sensitivity while drop in stress hormones at older ages can cause ↑ sensitivity) -menstrual cycle (sensitivity typically ↑ in follicular phase and ↓ in luteal phase) -pregnancy (typically ↓ sensitivity and higher insulin needs in weeks 12-36, leveling off prior to delivery, and then sharp ↑ sensitivity and decreased insulin needs after delivery)

If we find a situation consistently throws off our numbers, we can test more often or use a CGM to monitor our body's reaction. Then we can plan ahead to prepare for similar situations in the future. Because situations that change insulin sensitivity pop up regularly in managing T1D, we'll talk more about forming strategies to tackle them in Part III.

A Continuous Process

When a sub 2-hour marathon is achieved, there is no doubt runners will find ways to become even faster. Research will continue to produce information for more efficient training. Equipment will be better. Training methods more advanced. Runners will have the potential to go beyond the bounds of what we now consider impossible. But only if they stay hungry. To gain this potential, they must continuously seek out new information...learning and relearning about the task at hand.

In T1D, there is no telling how far knowledge and treatments will progress in the near future. Some of the world's smartest scientists and doctors are working in T1D research. The first artificial pancreas system has been approved. We are staring down insulin-producing cells. Faster-acting insulin. Countless management tools that will make our lives easier. Our momentum has only just started.

But even the newest breakthroughs are not sufficient to improve our control. They don't create the outcomes...we do. To make the most of the growing body of knowledge and resources, we also have to stay hungry—seeking out information, using it regularly, and then refreshing. This holds true from basic T1D facts through the latest advancements. Brushing up on the basics is especially important as a firm understanding allows us to better grasp newer, more complex information.

This is what many health professionals call "continued education" and it's essential for every person with T1D. Luckily, it's not as painful as it sounds and not that hard to find. In addition to books and publications, there are many websites dedicated to spreading knowledge in everything and anything T1D. A few of my favorites are listed in Resources.

With all that said, training doesn't stop at learning about the task at hand. People can know all there is to know about running and not have ever logged a single mile. Similarly, we can have all the T1D knowledge in the world, but for it to mean anything, we have to apply it. Strategizing helps us utilize our knowledge—both what we learn secondhand and through personal experience.

PART III

FORMING (AND REFORMING) STRATEGIES

Speaking hypothetically, what would happen if all marathon runners ditched their training plans and made only impromptu decisions throughout their training? Disaster. Absolute disaster. Sleeping through alarms. Skipping runs. Injuries—LOTS of injuries. Inadequate physical and mental endurance to make it through races. No improvement. No more world records. There's a reason this situation is only hypothetical.

Few lucky people may be able to fudge their way across a finish line after approaching training this way, but all good runners know it takes planning ahead and strategizing to achieve long-term success. Decisions made in the moment are rarely the best. Impulse and emotion can easily overcome logic. We take the easy way out instead of doing what we know will produce the best results.

Similarly, many people with T1D are very capable of good control. They are motivated, seek out continued education, and have all the resources they need. Yet they still don't see the improvements they would like. Why? Because good management in theory and good management in practice are two very different things.

Knowledge isn't meant to sit in our heads. It's meant to transform our actions. Knowledge gives us the *potential* for better results, but those results only become reality when we use what we learn to proactively plan the actions we'll take to improve our management. Strategies form the bridge between the knowledge that creates potential and the actions that create results.

Yet out of any part of management, forming strategies tends to be what people gloss over the most. It was certainly underutilized in my own care growing up. And it's fairly easy to see why—forming strategies can be intimidating. Many people dismiss strategizing due to fear of not doing what's "right." But really, there is no one, "right" set of strategies for improving management...there are many!

In running, the best training strategy is whatever gets a runner across the finish line in one piece. My training plan to run Lake Placid was nothing like the one to run Boston. And my plan to run Boston probably didn't match the 30,000 training plans of the other runners.

In T1D, the best strategies are the ones that get us in range. These strategies change over time and are different from person to person. The only way we find what's best is by starting *somewhere*, and then tweaking as we learn.

Another barrier to forming strategies is the thought required up front. But over time, this small investment saves us a lot of hassle. It prevents in-the-moment contemplation, stress, and making excuses. It also prevents us from seconding-guessing whether or not we're doing enough in our care. Most importantly, because strategies are knowledge-based and molded by our own experiences, they maximize results while minimizing effort. Better control becomes easier to achieve.

Appropriately, my system for forming strategies developed from what I use to run marathons. It tackles two components of training: building skills and breaking down obstacles.

Building Skills

As runners set their aims higher, they almost always have the same objective in mind: be faster. The objective remains constant because, well, runners can always be faster. But how?

There are a lot of skills that go into cutting time off one's pace—developing strength in key muscle groups, increasing cardiovascular fitness, fueling correctly, tweaking form, getting adequate rest—the list goes on and on. Runners build these skills by setting goals and forming strategies to reach them. By improving in any one skill, they become closer to a faster pace.

In T1D, we also have a constant objective: tighter control. NOBODY spends 100% of their lives in range. To get as close as we possibly can, we develop the skills that go into daily management, such as:

SMBG Testing
- ensuring a clean testing site
- testing 6-10 times a day§ (meeting the ADA's minimum recommendations outlined in Part II)

Logging and Reviewing Results
- maintaining a log (written or digital)
- downloading meter and/or CGM results
- going over results regularly to find trends (many people shoot for once a week or once a month)
- ensuring proper date and time settings on equipment for review accuracy

---

§ If using traditional monitoring methods.

- entering blood sugars into pump or logging system, even when they're not needed for correction

Insulin Administration
- bolusing before meals under appropriate conditions
- maintaining awareness of insulin context (when last dose was taken and how much is still active)
- developing strategies to adjust insulin
- rotating injection or pump sites
- eliminating bubbles in insulin prior to administration
- for MDI regimens:
    - staying consistent with timing of basal insulin
    - pausing after injection to ensure full doses are delivered
    - calculating bolus doses with precision

Meals
- maintaining awareness of serving size and carb counts by:
    - reading labels
    - looking up carb counts
    - measuring (even just once goes a long way)
- planning meals in advance to aid in proper bolus timing

Supply Upkeep
- reordering supplies
- insulin, meter, and strip storage (i.e., avoiding extreme temperatures)
- regularly changing lancets, needle tips, and/or infusion sets
- disposing of needles properly

- having up-to-date insulin, ketone test strips, and glucagon

Team Communication
- establishing an agreed-upon plan for communication with members of T1D support team
- practicing honesty and openness about results
- making doctors appointments
- having primary care doctor, endocrinologist, and CDE contact information
- having pharmacy and supply company contact information
- contacting the endocrinologist or CDE when:
    - basal/bolus needs adjusting (i.e., sick days)
    - uncertain of how to get back in range
    - large ketones are present

Emergency Preparedness
- carrying fast-acting glucose
- keeping a few bucks handy to buy glucose if needed
- having extra battery available for insulin pump
- wearing a medical ID
- checking for ketones
- having a backup plan (i.e., if pump or pen malfunctions) and extra supplies
- maintaining a written record of insulin:carb ratios, correction factors, and basal rates or dose
- teaching certain family members and friends how to use glucagon
- traveling prepared (this is especially important as travel often changes our routines drastically)
    - keeping a list of necessary supplies

- packing enough supplies (~2 times the amount we would normally need)
- packing supplies in carry-on luggage
- taking familiar snacks with known carb content (I usually go with protein bars and almonds)

Healthy Lifestyle
- making nutritious food choices
- participating in regular physical activity
- getting adequate sleep (recommendation = 8-10 hours for teenagers and 7-9 hours for adults 18+)[1]
- drinking enough water (recommendation = ~2.5-4 liters/day depending on age, sex, and physical activity)[2]

Endurance
- finding our supporters
- connecting with those in similar situations
- seeking rewards (both internal and external)
- developing mental strength
- living with purpose

*more to come on all of these topics in Part IV

    The list of T1D management skills is <u>long</u>. And thankfully, tighter control isn't a product of improving all of these skills at once but rather by working on any *one* of these skills, and then building them up over time. To do this, we set goals and form strategies to reach them.

    When I work on a skill, it helps me to think in terms of SMART. SMART is a memorable acronym that serves as goal and strategy guidance in all fields whether it be sports, business, or T1D. With several variations of SMART, here is a version I have found fitting for improving management skills: **S**pecific, **M**easurable, **A**s easy as possible, **R**ealistic, and **T**uned-in.

Specific

Goals are meant to be the smallest, most narrow workings of our training, yet they are often confused to be the broadest. "Tighter control" isn't a goal. Nor is "test blood sugar more often," "bolus earlier," so on and so forth. Goals shouldn't be grand and vague. Rather, goals should target a very specific action. Who does the action involve? What does it entail? When is it supposed to happen? Where will it take place? We should be able to paint a picture of ourselves making this change in our daily routines. For example, instead of "count carbs more often" we could choose "learn one carb count a day of a regularly-eaten food item using the CalorieKing app and screenshot for a total of 30 pictures this month."

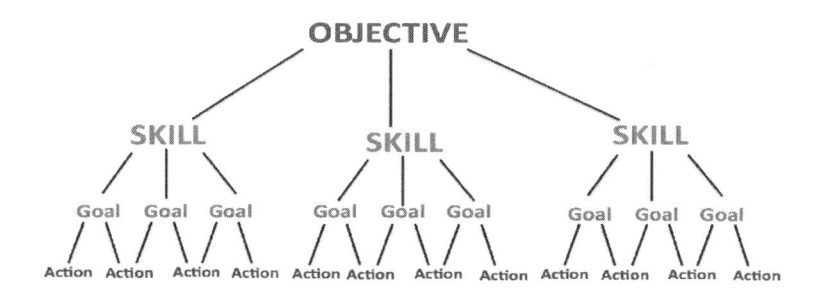

Our objective of tighter control is made up of skills. Skills are made up of goals and goals are made up of actions.

Measurable

Goals make use of concrete data. There should be no subjectivity or judgement involved—that only means extra work! We either follow through with an action or we don't.

Having a system to measure progress (i.e., check marks, numbers, or tallies) keeps us accountable and lets us know if we're meeting our goals. When we stay on track, we get the positive feedback we deserve. When we don't, we get an indicator that our strategies may need tweaking.

As Easy as Possible

If we thought the actions to meet our goals were easy, we'd be doing them already. Behind every change we would like to make are barriers—reasons that hold us back from doing what we know is best. "I always forget." "It takes too much time." "It's too far away." "I don't know how." We are 200% more likely to make changes if we proactively address our barriers. What can we do to make the action as easy as possible?

One way is by changing our environment. It's much easier to change our surroundings than change ourselves. By nature, we do what is most convenient. Want to use something more often? Make it close and easy to grab. Want to use something less often? Tuck it away somewhere hard to access (I use this method with junk food). And since most of us don't live by ourselves, creating an environment conducive to reaching our goals is usually a team effort. It depends on communication skills—we have to let others know what we are trying to achieve and how they can help make it happen.

For adopting *new* actions, using cues can be helpful. Pairing new actions to certain, existing parts of our daily or weekly routines has proven to be an effective way of making new actions seem more natural.[3] One example is changing out lancets with every pump site change, every basal injection, or every bolus injection (if you're super ambitious). For actions that are difficult to pair, it can help to create new cues. For example, marking specific days on our calendars or setting reminders on our smartphones. I found this especially helpful when changing out pump sites or checking the status of supplies.

Finally, once we identify our barriers, we can find resources to help tackle them. Using available tools and technology makes achieving our goals more effortless—apps to calculate bolus doses, pens that keep track of insulin context, meters that link to insulin pumps…if you can think of it, it probably exists (or maybe you're the next millionaire inventor, who knows?).

An endocrinologist, CDE, or even others with T1D who have faced similar barriers can offer useful guidance on available resources. Publications and websites for people with T1D also offer great assistance for learning what is available and helpful to others. A few of my favorites are found in Resources.

Realistic

No matter the number of past races, I start just about every training regimen thinking five miles seems like a long way to go. Most certainly in those first few weeks, I wouldn't be ready to go on a 26.2-mile run. I would probably end up with a serious injury or mental burnout from putting myself through that sort of trauma. Instead, 26.2 miles comes from adding length progressively…usually about a mile a week. This method gradually builds strength, endurance, and confidence.

In T1D, we build management skills like a runner builds mileage—one step at a time. Trying to change too much too soon will most likely lead to not trying at all. Instead of tackling all of our management skills at once, it's more effective to gradually build a strong foundation…usually focusing on one or two skills at a time. This makes reaching our goals more feasible. And with every goal achieved, we gain confidence that we can execute the actions required for good management, also called self-efficacy. Self-efficacy then helps us persevere when we work toward more lofty goals in the future.

Tuned-In

Meeting our goals is a highly personalized process. It works best when we are tuned-in with a) how goals fit into our bigger picture and b) how well our strategies are working. One of the easiest ways to do this is by writing out our goals and displaying them in a prominent place where we will see them every day. This makes them easier to prioritize and practically impossible to forget. I usually write my goals atop my day planner or print them on a SMART template, which can be downloaded at everystepcountstld.org.

Being tuned-in also works in tandem with being **M**easurable—it lets us know how well we're staying on track. We can stay tuned-in by reviewing our progress at regular intervals (such as the end of the week or the end of the month) and making notes on what seems to work and what doesn't. This is another reason why I find it helpful to work with a calendar or template.

It's impossible to expect a change in routine to be consistent 100% of the time…when reviewing our progress, it's about what we do *most* of the time. If we follow through ~75-80% of the time with no problems, we may be ready to tackle another goal. If we do not, we may need to tweak our strategies. Finding what works best individually is a continuous process because it adapts over time to fit our changing lifestyles and personalities. Just because our objective is constant doesn't mean our methods cannot be flexible.

All together, here is a SMART example I would have used for my younger self on MDI:

Skill: Calculating Bolus Doses

S- Perform math before lunch bolus at school using proper insulin:carb ratios and correction factors.

M- Check mark on template for every proper bolus calculation...keep template with insulin pen.

A- Barriers: 1) It takes too much time to do the math before every bolus. 2) Math is tedious and I don't have a smartphone for bolus dose calculations. Solution: make charts that correspond to insulin:carb ratios and correction factors to keep with template.

R- The only math I will have to do is adding if I am out of range and have a correction...that's extra incentive to be in range before lunch so I don't have to do the extra math.

T- This will improve my control because my blood sugars are inconsistent in the afternoon when I go to skating practice. I skate better in range. Plus, it's embarrassing to go to the endocrinologist and not know what insulin:carb ratios and correction factors I'm supposed to be using.

October SMART Skill: Bolus Calcs

S- perform math before lunch bolus at school using proper I:C ratios and correction factors.
M- check mark on template for every proper bolus calculation...keep template with insulin pen.
A- Barriers: 1) It takes too much time to do the math before every bolus. 2) Math is tedious and I don't have a phone for bolus dose calculations. Solution: make charts that correspond to I:C ratios and correction factors to keep with template.
R- The only math I will have to do is adding if I am out-of-range and have a correction...that's extra incentive to be in-range before lunch so I don't have to do the extra math.
T- This will improve my control because my blood sugars are inconsistent in the afternoon when I go to skating practice. I skate better in-range. Plus, it's embarrassing to go to the endocrinologist and not know what I:C ratios and correction factors I'm supposed to be using.

Sunday	Monday	Tuesday	Wednesday	Thursday	Friday	Saturday	Notes
	1 ✓	2 ✓	3 problem w/ lunch carb count...	4 ✓	5 ✓	6 ✓ home lunch	look at lunch menu ahead of time
7 brunch...skipped lunch	8 ✓	9 ✓	10	11	12	13	
14	15	16	17	18	19	20	
21	22	23	24	25	26	27	
28	29	30	31				

Insulin: Carb Ratio of 1:12	
Carbohydrates (g)	Insulin (units)
6	0.5
12	1.0
18	1.5
24	2.0
30	2.5
36	3.0
42	3.5
48	4.0
54	4.5
60	5.0
66	5.5

Correction factor of 1:70 w/ 130 target	
Blood glucose (mg/dL)	Additional Insulin (units)
165	0.5
200	1.0
235	1.5
270	2.0
305	2.5
340	3.0
375	3.5

Example of SMART template with checkboxes similar to my marathon training plans (see Part IV for Boston's) as well as insulin:carb ratio and correction factor charts. These templates can be found online at everystepcountst1d.org.

Other SMART examples I have used in the past include:

Skill: Wearing Medical ID

S- Consistently wear medical ID to class and on runs.

M- A check on my calendar the days I wear it, a check plus if I wear it the entire day.

A- Barriers: 1) Most of the IDs I've tried are clunky. 2) When I take them off, I forget to put them back on. Solution: ask people who consistently wear a medical ID what kind they use (RoadID ended up working really well).

R- I have worn jewelry consistently before, so I know this isn't unreasonable. I just have to find an option that fits an active lifestyle. Even wearing a medical ID sometimes is better than not wearing one at all.

T- Emergencies can happen to anyone and I don't go around with a medical ID tattoo—Mom would kill me! If something happens, people need to know. It also serves as proof of T1D to get food and drinks into movie theaters.

Skill: Reordering Supplies

S- Check amount and expiration date of T1D supplies on the first of every month. Reorder new and discard expired supplies if necessary.

M- One check mark by the month name on my calendar for every time I complete this task.

A- Barriers: 1) It takes time away from things I would rather be doing. Solution: give a time limit and set a timer…five minutes will be a good start. If it goes over, move to five minutes the next day. 2) Going over all of my supplies seems daunting. What if I forget to check some? Solution: make a list of supplies so I will not have to remember which need checking on the spot.

R- Five minutes out of 43,800 minutes a month isn't too much to ask.

T- Being proactive will help ensure that I will not be inconvenienced by unexpected supply issues. Knowing I went over supply status once a month is also better than worrying about it multiple times a month.

Breaking Down Obstacles

In addition to building up skills, runners can train to be faster by addressing the obstacles that slow them down. Hills, unfamiliar terrain, extreme weather, medical conditions like T1D…we are bound to face some sort of challenge *regardless* of skill level. By recognizing our obstacles, we can strategize and be more prepared to tackle them in the future.

In T1D, daily obstacles stand in the way of tighter control because, as we talked about in Part II, so many transient factors contribute to how our bodies react to a given amount of insulin. Even though our insulin regimen is based on our "normal" routines and physiology, our routines and bodies often stray from normalcy. With that said, we do tend to be creatures of habit. The obstacles we face are typically ones we are bound to see again—finding basal rates that work best with the start of school, the snack that puts us in range after a group fitness class, so on and so forth.

These obstacles manifest themselves in blood sugar trends. In range or out of range, blood sugars are never an accident. There are always reasons....we just have to find them. When do we tend to go out of range? What are the patterns? Trends are clues that help us pinpoint our obstacles and how me might tackle them. We can gather these clues in a few ways.

First, we can download blood sugars straight from our meters. Most meters come with software that displays blood sugars in daily, weekly, or monthly intervals. These downloads are our snapshots in time. Alternatively, CGMs give a more detailed story, including the times when we're not likely to test like after meals or when we're sleeping. Because CGMs give continuous tracings, trends are easier to see. Some CGM software even detects trends and suggests areas for improvement. Finally, we can use manual logging to track blood sugars using smartphone apps, or with old-fashioned pen and paper. Even if we only record out-of-range numbers and when they happen, this can be an incredibly useful tool.

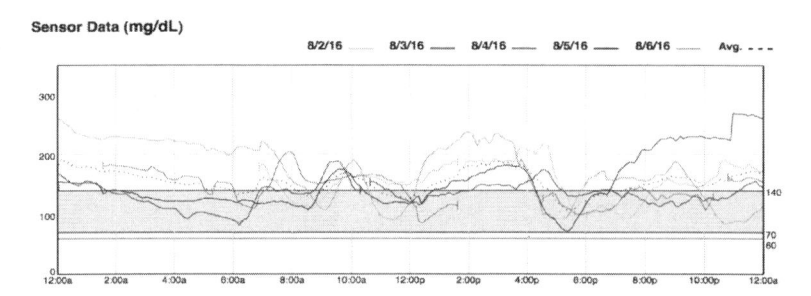

CGM tracing during a change in routine at work. These trends helped my endocrinologist and me to tweak my insulin regimen, lowering these post-meal spikes and overall average. *Image from Medtronic CareLink software.*

Each experience can be used to tailor our strategies. Since it's impossible to remember *every* combination of insulin, carbs, activity, and timing we've tried to stay in range, logging is extremely helpful. After my "not-Jamestown-Beach" incident when I figured out the hard way that taking guesses at insulin doses was unsafe, I made a log to keep track of the strategies I tried and how they worked. As my body became more adjusted to running over the years, I continued to use similar logs to keep track of pre, during, and post-run strategies.

By taking something away from every long run, my strategies became more tailored and my blood sugars more stable. While training for the Boston Marathon, my strategy for long runs ten miles or more was: wake up early, test, take 10-15% of my recommended bolus dose for a white bagel with cream cheese (50 carbs), and set a temporary basal of 5% about 15 minutes before the run. On the run, I would have a running gel (20 carbs) every eight miles and take 0.1 units. Finally, I would cancel my temporary basal with about a mile left to go and take a regular bolus for a banana, peanut butter, and Kashi cereal with almond milk (55 carbs).

BOSTON LOG

Starting Blood Sugar (mg/dl)	Time	Basal	Bolus	Carbs	Activity	Ending Blood Sugar (mg/dl)	Time	Notes
113	6:30am	5% 1 hour	Rec 3.75 → 11% = 0.4	50 bagel w/ 1 tbsp cream cheese	9 miles	161	8am	try 0.1 unit for 20c gel ↓
159	6:30am	" "	Rec 4.25 11% = ~0.5	" "	11 miles	126	8:15am	worked better ✓
130	4pm	" "	11% rec	20 1 cup plain Cheerios	8 miles	72	5:15pm	low @ mile 5. try 8% rec in PM
142	6:00am	5% 1.5 hours	" "	50 bagel w/ 1 tbsp cream cheese	14 miles	220	8:00am	forgot 0.1 for gel
105	6:00am	5% 2 hours	" "	" "	16 miles	128	8:15am	✓

Log entries in preparation for the Boston Marathon. This template can be found at everystepcountst1d.org.

I have also used logging for other situations dealing with school, work, cheerleading, travel, insulin adjustment, and even eating foods with mysterious nutritional content. Here's a recent example I used for the Medical College Admission Test (MCAT)—a 7-hour test where staying in range was essential to doing my best.

MCAT LOG

Starting Blood Sugar (mg/dl)	Time	Basal	Bolus	Carbs	Activity	Ending Blood Sugar (mg/dl)	Time	Notes
130	8:00am	normal	3.6	45 banana, coffee, cereal	3 hours practice test	250	11:00am	Do NOT do high G-I foods for breakfast or coffee... too many restroom breaks
160	8:00am	normal	2.7	30 apple, water, plain Greek yogurt	4 hours practice test	173	12pm	Try 1 hour temp basal & super bolus
108	8:00am	super bolus - temp ↓ basal	2.3 + 0.6 = 2.9	" "	5 hours practice test	150	1pm	try almonds for snacking
92	8:00am	" "	" "	" "	full practice! (7 hours)	115	3pm	✓
96	8:00am	" "	" "	" "	4 hours practice	111	12pm	✓

Logging also guided me to an effective strategy for the MCAT.

Because our bodies are constantly changing and adjusting to a changing environment, one common obstacle is basal/bolus adjustment. When there's no specific event or stimulus that happens before a trend, it may indicate that our insulin regimen needs some tuning up. When available, using insulin pump downloads in combination with a meter or CGM download helps us to see how basal rates and boluses correspond to our trends.

Since adjusting an insulin regimen can be complicated, it is always best to get the opinion of an endocrinologist or CDE. They can walk us through the steps to find appropriate basal rates, insulin:carb ratios, and correction factors. There are also additional professional resources to help us effectively adjust insulin such as the aforementioned *Pumping Insulin*.

However, at some point or another, we are bound to face unexpected obstacles we didn't have the chance to prepare for. SO many crazy things can happen in this world and we cannot waste time worrying about "what if…?" situations (we'll never be able to think of them all anyway). Instead, we can answer "what if…?" questions through preparation of what we can control, and then move on. This is where emergency preparedness comes into play as a management skill. By covering our bases (having fast-acting glucose, wearing our medical IDs, carrying extra supplies, etc.), we can prevent unexpected situations from getting dangerous.

Stepping Outside the Comfort Zone

By far, the biggest barrier that prevents people from finding the most effective management strategies is openness to trying new things. Again, for better or worse, we tend to be creatures of habit. We don't like change and it's easy to be close-minded when we're already comfortable with the way we manage our T1D. But what's *comfortable* may not be what's *best*. As the saying goes, "If you always do what you've always done, you'll always get what you've always gotten." If you have perfect blood sugars, by all means, don't change a thing! But if you don't (which is ~99.98% of us), being open to trying new things is key to finding the best management strategies. Without stepping outside the comfort zone, T1D would still be treated with strange diets. Plus, most things only seem mysterious and intimidating until we actually try them.

When trying new management strategies, it helps to:

Remember Nothing Is Set in Stone

New adjustments in our management are not permanent. Trying a new insulin reduction before exercise, a pump instead of MDI, a CGM or other new technology...anything! If it doesn't work after a fair shot, the old way will still be there. Nothing is lost. In fact, when adjustments don't work out, we gain assurance that our current strategies work better than new ones.

Be Systematic

As we talked about in Part II, insulin, carbs, and activity are the variables we control that drive blood sugars. When forming strategies, we should only change one variable at a time. If we change insulin, carbs, and activity all at once, we may not know which variable had the effect we wanted. For example, I kept my breakfast (both food and timing) consistent before long runs, but would change the % of recommended bolus. And when adjusting a single variable, we need to be systematic. No random guessing! For example, carbs or insulin should be adjusted by a % of normal or in concrete increments.

Be Conservative

Small changes are less intimidating than drastic ones, not to mention much safer—especially when there's insulin involved. It's better to start small, and then build up...not the other way around. As always, testing more often or using a

CGM is our best safeguard when facing unfamiliar situations or trying new management strategies.

Use Others' Knowledge and Experiences

Solving problems in daily management doesn't require us to be experts in anything and everything T1D. We aren't expected to know all possible strategies, resources, or science. But there are people who spend a good chunk of their lives trying—endocrinologists and CDEs. They get excited about boosting our management efforts and they're good at it. They help us form strategies, meet goals, and suggest areas for improvement we may not have thought of ourselves. In this marathon we live, endocrinologists and CDEs are our coaches. Their expertise is invaluable.

Another powerful resource is people who have been in similar situations. In marathon training, consulting runners who had already run the Boston Marathon helped prepare me for Heartbreak Hill—a steep hill that's half a mile long and placed about 20 miles into Boston's course.[4] At this point, runners are beyond fatigued, running on tired legs, and *still* have about six miles left to go. It's called Heartbreak Hill because runners so easily become disheartened by this perfect storm of physical and mental challenge.

Not having any comparable hills to train on in Williamsburg, VA, I was terrified. If I didn't prepare somehow, my heart was the one that would be broken on Heartbreak Hill. I needed ideas, so I hunted down other Boston marathoners from Williamsburg to see how they trained. The answers? Wall sits, planks, and resistance bands to build strength in key muscle groups. Incline bouts on the treadmill. Plyometrics for explosive power. Losing 10 lbs.

It was obvious that some of those suggestions needed to be taken with a grain of salt (losing 10 lbs would not have been healthy for a small-framed girl!). However, their advice gave me a great starting point. I picked certain suggestions to add to my training regimen and fine-tuned them over time to fit my needs. In the end, trying those new strategies made me a stronger runner. And when the moment finally came to run Heartbreak Hill, I didn't even realize I was running it until I saw other runners starting to walk and a sign: "Congratulations, you conquered Heartbreak Hill!" Pretty anticlimactic, I know…but it means I must have been very prepared!

One nice thing about T1D is that even though we are all unique in our personal races, we run the same course and can share ideas about the obstacles we face. Suggestions from others can act as starting points for our own strategies, even if we don't necessarily think we'll take them. For example, you may discover that you despise thinking in terms of SMART or using a written log. These strategies (for forming strategies) may not work for you and that's totally fine! Either way, you will learn more about your own likes and dislikes by trying, which will take you one step closer to finding a system that works best for you. There is no absolute right or wrong. Whatever is effective and you are most likely to maintain is right for *you*.

Every day we gain personal, trial-and-error experiences that cannot be taught to us by anyone else. Every day offers opportunities to optimize our strategies…but only when we reflect to take something away. What worked and what did not? The more we pick up on the strategies that result in in-range numbers and repeat them, the more confidence we gain in daily management decisions. And as we practice forming strategies, our problem solving skills continue to evolve. Thinking of new solutions becomes easier. Strategies become more tailored to our bodies, our lifestyles, and where we are personally in our care. We spend more time in range.

But even with great strategies, deciding to execute the actions for effective management is not easy—it takes an *incredible* amount of discipline. The final part of this marathon approach focuses on the ability to carry out those actions over time. For this, we require endurance.

PART IV

BUILDING ENDURANCE TO GO THE DISTANCE

"The race is not won to the swift, nor the strong, but to he who endures in the end."

-Ecclesiastes 9:11

Success in running, or anything in life for that matter, doesn't happen in an instant. It takes time. Sometimes, a long time. And along the way, success isn't linear. In some weeks of training, runners clock in record times. 18-mile runs don't seem all that grueling. Runners see hard work pay off and it encourages them to work even harder. Other weeks, they are sick or battling injuries. Running hurts. At times, runners are unexplainably slower than usual.

Without the feeling of progress, it's easy to ask "why bother?" and become discouraged. My marathon training was no exception. It had its ups and downs. Runner's highs followed by persistent low blood sugars. Record times followed by injuries. Some low points made me wonder if the sacrifices and pain of training were even worth it.

Now, I can look back and see that those low points taught me lessons that led to the high points. I became smarter about my training and got faster with every race. But in the moment, I could have easily concluded that my setbacks meant it wasn't possible to get any faster...to conclude that I had reached my limit and working harder wouldn't change my results. Deciding to ease up on training during low points would have been the easiest thing to do. But it also would have been a mistake.

Similar feelings are common in T1D. Management is the hardest training we will ever do. It's a 24/7 job that requires full attentiveness...everything we do and are exposed to affects our blood sugars. Even when we strive to make the right decisions, we can end up out of range. Sometimes, we just can't make sense of it all.

It would be nice to be just a little bit better every day...to always have tangible proof of our hard work. But that's not how it goes. Just like marathon training, the path to success is winding. The only guarantee is that there are bound to be setbacks, off-days, and plateaus. There will always be situations beyond our control. Of course it's normal to be knocked down at times and feel like our best isn't good enough. And in these moments when things aren't going our way, we are most tempted to take the easy way out....to ease up on our efforts or even give up altogether.

So how do we find the endurance to get past the bad times that catapult us into new personal bests? Two sources that I have found key are support and mental strength. The rest of this chapter takes a look at how each builds endurance.

<u>Support</u>
From those on the sidelines

The Boston Marathon is always held on the third Monday in April. A day popularly referred to as "Marathon Monday." And the weekend before, there are many long-standing city traditions...one being the "Blessing of the Athletes" at Old South Church—a beautiful, historic church with Gothic architecture situated right by the marathon's finish line on Boylston Street.

The memory of going to Blessing of the Athletes was as special as crossing the finish line. The energy was electric. The church was packed with a sea of runners and their supporters gathering together from all over the world to celebrate the Lord...and pray they'd be crossing the finish line the following day. Colorful ribbons waved high in the air as the Olympic Anthem played.

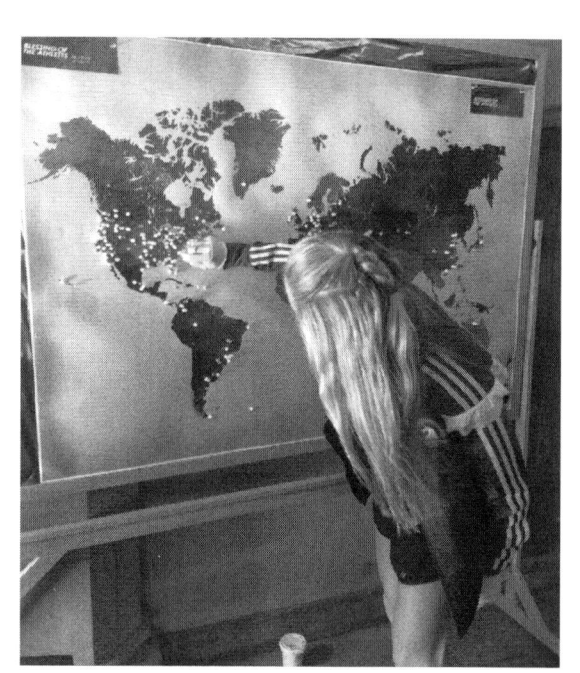

Runners and their supporters came from hundreds of countries, each represented by pushpins on a world map at the church's entrance.

Sun streamed in through elaborate stained glass windows that went up the entire length of the church's towering walls.

The theme of the service was molded around Ecclesiastes 9:11: *"The race is not won to the swift, nor the strong, but to he who endures in the end."* The pastor started by discussing what makes the Boston Marathon the most famous race in the world. She noted that the course itself doesn't stand out...it's not the easiest but certainly not the hardest. It wasn't the location (although I personally think Boston is pretty spectacular).

Instead, the pastor claimed the reason for Boston's legacy was "the spectators who are as celebrated as the race itself and part of the legend." The 500,000 people cheering us on along the sidelines who make the race possible to endure.

She had done the math: 500,000 spectators divided by 30,000 runners gave each runner a 17-person personal cheering section—a number she claimed was even greater than Justin Bieber's entourage. 17 people yelling a runner's name at the top of their lungs as he or she pushed past the hills. 17 people who thought the world of a runner, no matter the ultimate results. *They* were the ones who set the Boston Marathon apart.

Even when runners felt like the race was too much to handle, when they were scared, when they were tempted to give up—all of which the pastor was confident would happen at some point in the race—she urged, "Runners, you do not run this race alone."[1]

On race day, her sermon couldn't have held more true. The weather was 40 °F and raining, with winds over 20 mph. A runner's worst nightmare. At times my eyes were forced shut as the wind blew in rain from the opposite direction. Yet despite the horrendous conditions, there they were from start to finish—all 500,000 spectators. And they were *excited*. They knew they were needed. They were throwing high fives, holding signs, giving out snacks, offering towels, providing first aid...even kissing runners in some cases (looking at you, Wellesley girls). They offered inspiration, distraction, and relief. They reinforced the belief that the finish line would actually be there...and that it would be worth it.

None of the runners were listening to music, but even if we were, we wouldn't have been able to hear it because our spectators—our personal cheering sections of 17—were cheering so loudly. When I made the final turn onto Boylston Street toward the finish line, the cheers turned into a collective roar. I will probably never know what it's like to win a gold medal at the Olympics, but I can only imagine that's what it would sound like.

Every step of the way, when runners started feeling pain or fatigue...when we felt like giving up, all we had to do was look to those on the sidelines. Certainly, we were not running the race alone.

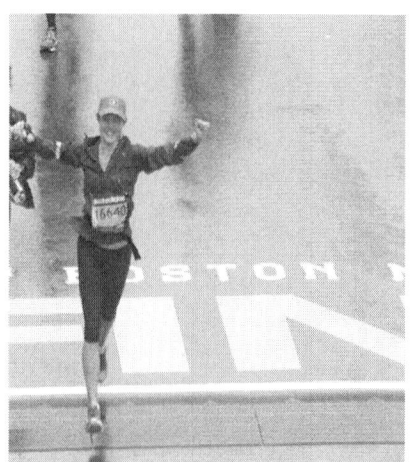

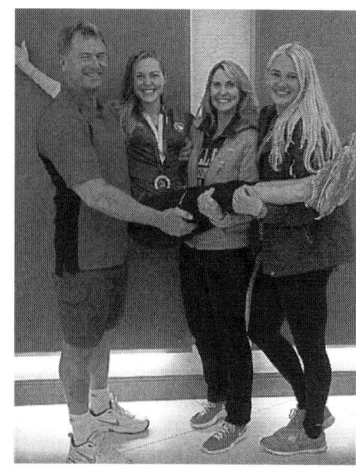

I was so overcome with emotion turning onto Boylston Street — everything I had worked for culminated in that one moment of crossing the finish line. My family's constant support was instrumental in reaching this goal and every goal.

Even though it can be difficult to recognize, our personal cheering section—this INCREDIBLE source of endurance—exists in the lives we lead every day with T1D. They are our family, friends, doctors, and mentors. They get us through the tough stuff and T1D management is no exception.

Not even the most disciplined person with T1D can go at it alone. While we don't need a 17-person entourage, we need at least a few other people to relieve the burden of T1D and help us reach our maximum potential. Besides giving us high fives for in-range numbers and tossing us glucose tabs when we're low, our supporters can:

Listen

Even if there's nothing someone else can do to help change a situation, the act of listening can be equally as powerful. When people listen to what we have to say, they're giving us their most precious gifts: time and attention. Listening is a way of saying, "I am here to learn about what you're going through. To feel what you're feeling. To be there for you in any way I can."

Opening up about our experiences is beneficial to our relationship with anyone in our T1D support team. Others feel trusted and have the opportunity to relate to us on a deeper level. We gain comfort and validation that our hardships are not trivial. Talking things out can even help us reframe problems and move forward with new energy.

Give Encouragement

One of my favorite things during a race is high fives from kids on the sidelines. With eager faces, they wait for runners to pass by. With every "hit," they get so excited...like they are the ones receiving the favor. Little do they know they are doing more for the runner than the runner is doing for them.

When I get a high five, a "good job," or a "looking strong," I'm boosted. My pace gets faster and the pain temporarily subsides. That single event replays in my mind for miles.

In running and T1D, a little encouragement goes a long way. Even if we know it to be true, it's nice to have a reminder that what we do isn't easy and we're doing a good job.

Encouragement is so important that there are award programs to honor the hard work we put in day in and day out. These external rewards are great gateways to the internal rewards of better T1D control. Some awards include the Lilly Diabetes Journey Award and the Joslin Medalist Program. Milestones for both awards include 25, 50, and 75 years lived with T1D while Lilly Diabetes also has a 10-year award. For teens and young adults, there are also multiple scholarships available, including one that proceeds from this book support: the Every Step Counts Scholarship Program. Information about these awards and scholarships are listed in Resources.

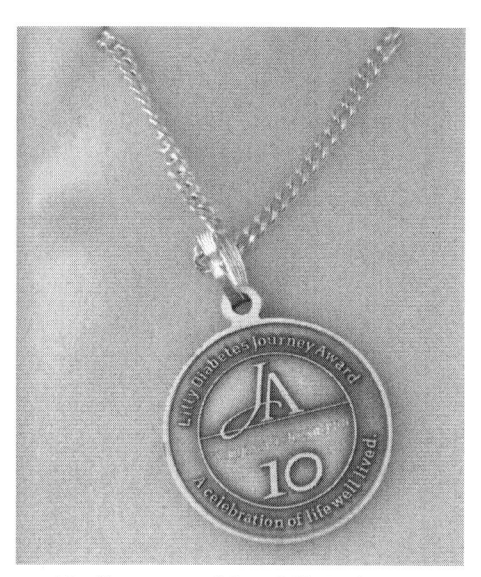

My 10-year award from Lilly Diabetes is a great reminder that what I do every day matters and to keep working hard.

Lend a Fresh Perspective

When we're emotionally invested in a situation, it can be hard to remove ourselves and see the objective reality. As a runner who was used to training in a relatively mild climate, seeing the 40 °F, rainy, and windy weather forecast for the day of the Boston Marathon made me uneasy. Unless you're Meb Keflezighi in Chorale 1, most runners wait outside for hours before their chorale is called to the starting line. And then there's the additional 3 hours of outdoor running. My head was spinning with all the things that could possibly go wrong within that ~5 hour timespan. Hypothermia. Stiff muscles. A watery death for my pump and meter.

My family and friends helped calm me down and keep things in perspective—this wasn't the first time people raced in these conditions. I needed to stay solution-focused instead of wasting energy ruminating on hypotheticals.

My friend Carly reassured me, "There's no such thing as bad weather, only bad gear and bad attitudes." I could fix my attitude…but what about the gear?

My mom and I asked for advice from more experienced runners and were instructed to get "throwaways"—pieces of clothing worn for warmth and then given away for donation prior to the race. We settled for some sweatpants from the little boy's section of a department store (as you can tell, we had a difficult time finding something appropriate) and some oversized gloves. Warmth, check! Now for the rain and wind. Our solution? A plastic poncho and trash bags with holes for arms. Ziplock bags for my pump and meter.

Truth be told, I didn't want to go to the biggest race of my life in trash bags and little boy's sweatpants. When I saw how silly it looked, I insisted that I would be fine without them. But my mom wouldn't let me leave before I was thoroughly wrapped in plastic. With extra trash bags…just in case.

When I got to the race, never had I been so happy to look so ridiculous. I was warm. I was dry. Many runners were not. I made friends by giving away those extra trash bags. In return, these new friends offered invaluable advice about the course and helped guide me to the right place for my starting chorale. When it came time to run, I stripped off everything except one yellow poncho over my running clothes and was good to go.

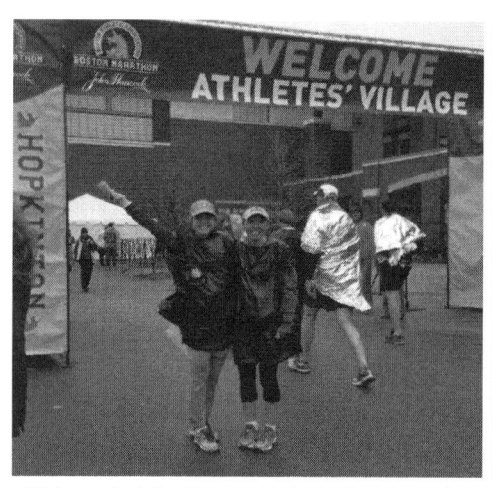

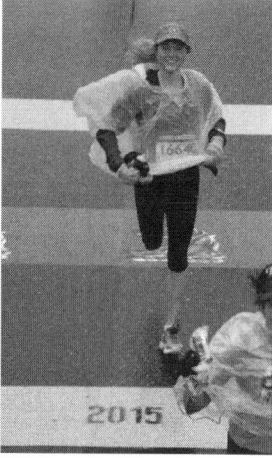

With my foolish…I mean fool proof outfit (and matching friends), I was ready to run. The yellow poncho stayed on until mile 20!

T1D is not something we take lightly (I know that to be true because otherwise you wouldn't have made it this far in the book). It's only natural that we are emotionally invested. And it's not a bad thing. However, this investment can sometimes hamper our problem solving skills. To be our best, we need people who can offer fresh ideas and help us step outside our own point of view to handle situations with a clear mind. Even if they don't have T1D themselves, those involved in our care—family, friends, significant others, and of course, doctors and CDEs—all have that ability.

Create a Conducive Environment

In college, sometimes the environment is not the most conducive to marathon training. Some nights, I was up until the wee hours of the morning because of neighbors' house parties and then had to wake up at 6 a.m. for a run. I was sometimes the party pooper for making smart choices…saying no to late nights, drinks, and other junk that my friends were having. All of which was fine. They could have a different lifestyle because they weren't trying to do what I was trying to do. But not having a mutual understanding sometimes made training a lot harder than it needed to be.

When people understand our goals, they'll create an environment to help us achieve them. These are our supporters. With T1D, they are on board with our aim of tighter control. They know the time and attention needed for T1D care are huge. Thus, supporters help create an environment that makes T1D care a top priority.

They encourage us to take care of ourselves properly without feeling like we're missing whatever else is going on. Whether it's pausing to test our blood sugar, having the time we need to calculate a proper bolus dose, or getting information to help estimate carbs in a home-cooked meal.

Creating a conducive environment also means having access to essential T1D supplies like insulin and test strips as well as other tools like healthy foods and fast-acting glucose. If we have the resources we need, we are infinitely more likely to succeed. Without adequate resources, living with T1D is impossible. Having our supporters on the same page makes life a lot easier—not having to constantly advocate for the necessities that come with T1D is a huge blessing.

Keep Us Accountable

People have different ways of staying accountable—following through with the actions required to meet their goals. Some people feel most motivated with self-tracking while others feel more responsible for their actions when they know someone else will be checking in. There is no right or wrong. It all depends on the person and goal.

For example, when it comes to running, I follow through on my own using techniques like my training spreadsheet. Having others check in to see if I completed my workouts would become an annoyance. Alternatively, someone may only be able to work out when they know they're meeting up with a friend.

If we have tried to keep ourselves accountable without much luck, engaging someone in our T1D support team may be a good call. But to do this effectively, it needs to be decided in advance. The middle of an argument is not the ideal time to start collaborating. It also must be done with mutual understanding. How will this person keep us accountable? When will they do it? Are there rewards? Are their consequences? And of course, we need open, honest communication with this person. Here's an example:

In high school, I had issues remembering if I had taken my long-acting insulin in the morning because it had become so routine (it was also early in the morning and I was half-asleep). To keep me accountable, my mom would ask if I remembered to take it…as I was getting out of the car for school. This really caused some friction as I kept my long-acting insulin at home. If I had forgotten, it would be too late to do anything about it. And walking into school, I was much more concerned with making a good impression on my peers than I was with my insulin. We were rightly using teamwork to keep me on track, but going about it the wrong way.

Luckily, we were enrolled in a study that aimed to improve child/parent communication in T1D management. It was in the study that we learned accountability works best for <u>both</u> parties when there is an agreement of how it will work. So we decided I would shout, "I'm taking my insulin!!!" and if my mom didn't hear it, she could ask me at the door before we walked out of the house. This worked much better than good intentions alone and saved a lot of frustration.

Other accountability ideas include predetermined text reminders or monetary rewards for every time a behavior is executed (which has actually been shown to increase positive management habits and improve results in young adults with T1D).[2]

Offer Inspiration

Even unknowingly, others can give us endurance to keep working hard solely through their own example. It may sound silly, but when someone else achieves a new personal record, I want one, too! I start thinking about my next race and get excited for training. Seeing a runner go out in bad weather, I think, "if they can handle the rain, snow, wind, etc., so can I!" The people who inspire us can be those we interact with on a daily basis, celebrities, or total strangers. Inspiration is found everywhere in anyone who pushes us to be better versions of ourselves.

In T1D, I tend to be inspired by those living with any chronic condition. One person in particular is the late Sam Berns, who was born with a genetic disorder called progeria. This condition causes premature aging. As Sam mentions in his TED Talk "My Philosophy for a Happy Life," the disorder affects only about 350 children in the entire world. At the age of 17, he weighed a fragile 50 lbs yet found ways throughout his life to achieve his dreams with a simple, three-part philosophy: "...all in all, I don't waste energy feeling bad for myself (1). I surround myself with people that I want to be with (2) and I keep moving forward (3)."[3] Listening to people like Sam, it's impossible not to feel recentered and motivated.

Support
From those who share the same course

As impressive as a 17-person entourage seems, the pastor at Old South Church underestimated each runner's true number of supporters by a modest 30,000. She was missing the other runners. Besides our matching Adidas Boston race jackets, runners shared in the early morning alarms, winter runs in sub-freezing temperatures, joy of qualifying, and triumph of pushing our boundaries. We established a camaraderie through the "been there, done that" of training. By default, we were invested in each other's Boston Marathons because we knew how much it took to get there.

That's why it's not uncommon to see runners helping other runners cross the finish line when they're injured. Or hear words of encouragement in desolate places along the race course. Every step of the journey, we are each other's support.

In T1D, we run this race together. We share a bond of common experiences and are never alone in the problems we face. We relate to each other on a much deeper level than anyone else can.

Similar to those on the sidelines, supporters with T1D have the ability to:

- listen,
- give encouragement,
- lend a fresh perspective,
- create a conducive environment,
- keep us accountable, and
- offer inspiration.

But they also have the in-depth understanding of all that goes into T1D physically, mentally, and socially...not only what can be observed or communicated. *They just know.*

They've shared in our frustrations and know what to say when we're discouraged. They give sound advice because it comes from a place of valuable, real-life experience. They know the environment and resources we need because they need them, too. They can be held accountable

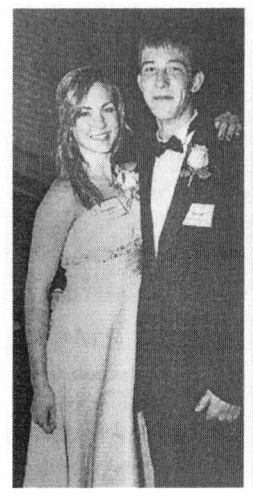

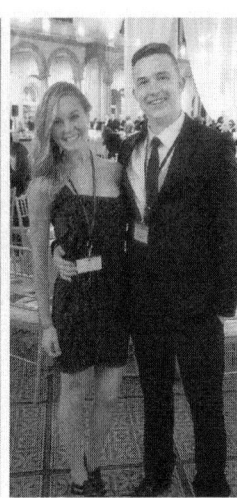

My best friend, David, and I met at JDRF's Night of Hope Gala in high school as youth ambassadors (left). After graduating from college, we now lead the youth ambassadors at the annual galas in D.C. and Baltimore.

with us because they want to improve their control just like we do. They continuously inspire us to work harder through their out-of-this-world accomplishments, augmented by solid control. Research has even shown that connecting with others who have T1D has the power to improve A1Cs in teens and young adults.[4] The support we give to each other is irreplaceable.

Since diagnosis, my entryway to the T1D community has been through involvement in JDRF (formerly the Juvenile Diabetes Research Foundation). Personally, JDRF helped my family and me with the coping process and even today, offers useful resources for camaraderie and continued education. In the past 14 years with T1D, I have met lifelong friends through JDRF and have had the opportunity to give back through volunteering, mentoring, and speaking as a professional athlete with T1D. I learn from every interaction with others who have T1D, their families, and their care teams. These encounters have made me better both as a person and as a person living with T1D.

There are plenty of opportunities to join organizations like JDRF nationally and internationally. Additionally, there are camps, local support groups, and online sites for people with T1D to connect. Some examples of each are listed in Resources.

Sharing the Race

Going back to our hypotheticals, what would happen if the Boston Marathon were run inside a dark, concrete tunnel instead of out in the open? Supporters on the sidelines would have no idea what was going on. Any encouragement would be lost. High fives gone. Cheers wasted. They would have no way of knowing how to help. Even worse, runners inside the tunnel would start to feel isolated….like they were running the race alone. It sounds like a long, miserable 26.2-mile nightmare.

Yet in life with T1D, it can be easy to create this concrete tunnel around ourselves and make our race harder than it has to be. We don't express our needs or our goals. We shut out potential supporters because we're afraid of judgement….that we may suffer embarrassment or disappoint others by showing our imperfections.

These notions are not facts, but rather untrue assumptions. They only serve to prevent us from having open, honest communication and getting the support we need. Nobody is perfect…not even close. Our supporters know that. When trying our best, the only time we face judgment from people who want to help us is when they don't understand enough about our situation and simply need to learn. After all, our supporters are not mind readers and the nuances of T1D can be hard to understand, especially if you don't live with it yourself. Because our supporters want to help us, they *want* to learn. The more we teach them about our needs and goals, the easier it becomes for them to share in our race.

First and foremost, this requires good communication—a willingness to be open about what we experience and the patience to explain information we take for granted. Good communication is a high-yield skill that we can build up over time and it applies to relationships with any member of our T1D support team.

Additionally, supporters boost our endurance by giving us extra motivation: we owe it to them and we owe it to ourselves to continuously strive to be better. And they help make it possible. With our supporters, we achieve personal bests beyond what we could ever achieve on our own.

At the end of the day, however, others can only help us as much as we let them. As the old saying goes, "You can't help someone who doesn't want to help themselves." Before we can effectively share our race, we first have to be in the right frame of mind to tackle the challenges of living with T1D. Other people can certainly help fuel our endurance, but ultimately it has to come from within. Thus, we work to develop the highest-yield skill in T1D: mental strength.

Mental Strength

In every race, there will inevitably be very capable runners who stop running before they reach the finish line. Even though their bodies can go farther….even though they have all the support….the resources, the encouragement, the inspiration that an athlete could ever want…they stop. Simply because that's what their minds are made up to do.

Runners will quit when the going gets tough if they do not develop mental strength along with physical strength. Without it, even the most talented, well-supported people fail to reach their full potential.

Mental strength is essential in running and even MORE so in life with T1D. We see setbacks happen daily. We have blood sugars that make no sense. Our results are a constant reminder that everything we do and are exposed to affects our bodies (no pressure, right?). Yet we have to stay level-headed. As Sam Berns laid out in his philosophy, we must *keep moving forward*.

Mental strength is not something we're born with, but rather a skill that is developed with practice. We enhance or diminish mental strength every day by the way we think. We can't always control what happens, but we do control our reactions and our thoughts. In both running and T1D, practicing a positive mindset and finding a sense of purpose are vital for building the mental strength to get through temporary setbacks.

Positive Mindset

> *"Your beliefs become your thoughts,*
> *Your thoughts become your words,*
> *Your words become your actions,*
> *Your actions become your habits,*
> *Your habits become your values,*
> *Your values become your destiny."*

-Mahatma Gandhi, renowned peace activist

The mind can be our biggest asset or worst enemy. In any situation life throws our way, we choose to react with one of two mindsets: positive or negative. One of these choices has the power to make our situation better while the other guarantees to make it worse.

My favorite runner of all time, Forrest Gump, demonstrates this concept beautifully on his months-long run across the United States. As the most famous runner of his time (at least he is in the movie), Forrest is running along when he is approached by a struggling entrepreneur looking for a new bumper sticker slogan.

As the two chat, Forrest accidentally runs through a big pile of dog poo. The whole time, Forrest is completely unfazed. Never skips a beat. The entrepreneur is noticeably shocked, to which Forrest matter-of-factly responds "it happens."

The moral of the story: Forrest didn't let a small setback get him down. Unhampered, he kept on his mission to run across the country. And he succeeded. The entrepreneur was so moved, in fact, that Forrest even inspired a new slogan in the process!

Running into a pile of poo, racing in bad weather, unexpected blood sugars…"it happens."** On any given day, we can't control what happens to us, but we can control how we react through our choice of mindset.

Despite its obvious benefit, choosing a positive mindset isn't always as easy as it sounds. Nobody (not even Forrest Gump) approaches all challenges with optimism. Maintaining a positive mindset is incredibly difficult. Pulling ourselves back when we drift toward negativity takes practice.

Here are a few tools I've found helpful for maintaining a positive mindset in both running and T1D:

Remembering…

- What we're doing *right*
  When we're constantly trying to find areas for improvement, it's easy to focus on what we're doing wrong and forget all the things we're doing right. And there are many! We're doing a good job. Yes, we are always trying to be better, but in-range numbers are no accident. We did something right (likely *many* things right) to get there.

  So what are they? Give yourself a pat on the back. Write yourself a thank-you note! And if you need more proof, keeping track of progress (i.e., the check marks mentioned in Part III) helps us see the good things we're doing every day. Recognizing what we're doing right also boosts accountability. By seeing the effort we've already put in, we feel responsible to keep following through on the promises we make to ourselves.

** The PG version of the entrepreneur's bumper sticker slogan.

- Nothing is permanent
Too often when bad things happen, they get blown out of proportion. Isolated incidents get extended to future events, or worse, to who we are as people. *"I couldn't complete that workout. Guess I'm not cut out for it." "My blood sugars are always high when I wake up. I just can't figure it out."*

Even writing these statements is painful. First, setbacks happen to everyone. They just do. Second, we can't take setbacks personally when we're trying our best. Moments are just those—moments. We have thousands every day and each one is new. While characterizing moments in time can help us become better in the future, overgeneralizing will only tear us down. Moments are not permanent, end-all-be-all reflections of our lives.

Some tools that have been especially useful in avoiding this sort of false permanency are two important words. One word of time-specificity: "today." And one word of growth: "yet." *"I couldn't complete that speed workout today. I'm not strong enough yet." "I woke up with a high blood sugar today. I haven't figured it out yet."*

Everyone has something they could have done better today and something they haven't been able to do yet. These two words help turn our focus to how we can change things in the future rather than ruminate on the past.

These ideas are famously described by what motivation and psychology researcher, Dr. Carol Dweck, coined as a "growth mindset." She explains this mindset further in her TED Talk: "The Power of Believing That You Can Improve" and book: *Mindset: The New Psychology of Success*.[5]

- How we feel *afterwards*

  It seems as though many of life's decisions follow a certain pattern: ones that are more compelling in the moment often tear us down later on while more difficult decisions provide us with lasting satisfaction. When faced with tasks we don't want to do—whether it's going on a 6 a.m. training run or taking the time to order new T1D supplies—reminding ourselves beforehand of how we feel afterwards helps us to follow through. We can walk a little taller the rest of the day, taking pride in the fact that we accomplished something important. When we feel that empowerment, we gain the confidence that pulls us to make those same good decisions in the future.

- Just because it's important doesn't mean it has to be serious

  I would be lying if I said running for hours on end doesn't ever get tedious. Sometimes it seems like long runs will never end. And the more you think about how long it's taking, the longer it feels. To get through training runs, I would use mental games to entertain myself. Seeing how long I could go without looking at my running watch. Counting the blue cars only. Picking focus spots in the distance to run to. It seems small, but these silly games kept me from getting bored.

  While long runs may seem like they'll never end, T1D management actually never ends. It can be tedious and boring at times, but playing games can help keep us entertained and on track. How many in-range blood sugars can we get in a row? Can we guess carb values before looking them up? Making management a source of entertainment can be just the "reset" button we need to keep from getting tired of doing the same things over and over.

- The benefits
Because there's a long period of time between the initial excitement of signing up for a race and crossing a finish line, it can be easy to lose sight of the enthusiasm that inspired training in the first place. In T1D, endocrinology appointments are like our race days. Around this time, we start to realize what we do every day has a real, tangible impact. And for better or worse, it shows in our A1Cs. But months of time separate appointments and it can be easy to forget all the reasons why we work to improve our control. Therefore, we have to remind ourselves. As we go through our days we can ask, "How do in-range blood sugars help what I'm doing right now?" Guaranteed, there will be an answer. And of course, we can refresh ourselves by re-reading the list of daily and long-term benefits in Part I.

- We aim for progress, not perfection
Whether it's contemplating a quick three-mile run on a busy day or changing out a lancet, the same question has crossed my mind: "If I can't do it *all* the way or *all* the time, why should I do it now?" But it's this kind of thinking that closes the door to forming better habits. Training isn't an all-or-nothing. Every step counts and some is always better than none. By doing things *sometimes*, they eventually become more natural. It can also led to the realization that some management tasks are not as difficult or time consuming as they seem. We shouldn't miss open opportunities. And on that note…

Taking Advantage of the Times We CAN

When I don't fill in a check mark on my marathon training plan for a particular day, I write the specific reason why I wasn't able to do so. The reasons are few, but pretty entertaining...traveling to the Philippines, getting sick with food poisoning, a fugitive on the loose (true story). All were situations I truly had no control over.

I kept those rare situations in mind before training runs that I *could* do, but wasn't particularly excited about: "Because I don't know exactly what will happen in the future, I need to take advantage of this opportunity <u>now</u> when I know I <u>can</u>."

In T1D, we also face similar, uncontrollable situations that prevent us from practicing management skills the way we plan to. Mystery foods with questionable carb counts. Faulty machinery. Inability to plan ahead. We can only do our best with the conditions we're given. However, the number of out-of-the-ordinary situations is relatively small compared to those of our normal routines. Most of the time, we are able to follow through…it's just a matter of if we prioritize management or not.

Every box has a check mark, recorded change to my original plan (i.e., switching days of my long run), weekly totals, and reasons why training days were not completed.

It's the majority of what we do that creates better control. Life's unpredictability is extra motivation to create a future safety net by following through with every opportunity that we know we CAN.

Avoiding the Tendency to Compare

At the start of a race, you can't help but size up the runners around you. *"His warm up routine is so intense...he's probably a better runner than me." "Dang! Look at her muscles...I should have done more calf raises." "Everyone is so serious and fit...do I really belong here?"*

Even in T1D, it's easy to start thinking *"Look at how happy and healthy they are...they must have better control than I do."*

Looking from the outside in, we can see how ridiculous this sounds….yet we all do it: comparing how we feel on the inside to how others appear on the outside. But everyone, no matter his or her appearance, has insecurities when it comes to T1D. We all experience highs and lows. Good moments in management and not-so-good moments. We all run the same race under different conditions. The only person we can fairly compare ourselves to is, well, ourselves. By trying to be better than our previous selves, we move forward. By trying to be better than someone else, we go nowhere.

Using Self-Awareness

At any given moment of the day, there's a voice inside our heads providing a constant stream of inner dialogue.

On a run: *"I wonder what I'll have for breakfast…" "Oh wow, I like his sneakers." "Dog!" "Darn it, a hill."*

In T1D: **Wakes up* "Okay, time to test." "It's been 15 minutes since I've bolused right? Nine? Okay, close enough." "Extra P.E. today…I hope I didn't overdo it on the insulin." "Man, I need to change my pump site."*

Sometimes this voice runs away on its own, negative agenda…amplifying the bad and drowning out the good. And sometimes this voice (incorrectly) believes it has superpowers. Reading minds. *"My endocrinologist thinks I'm lazy because my A1C went up."* And predicting the future. *"Why try anything new? My blood sugars will be out of whack anyway."*

Left unchecked, our heads can quickly fill with negative, distracting assumptions about what others think of us, our future, and ourselves. It takes conscious effort to quiet this crazy voice and return ourselves to productive thinking. We do that by practicing self-awareness.

The first step is simply observing our thoughts without judgement…identifying negative thoughts while also accepting that they are natural. We can then remedy these negative thoughts in two ways:

1) Reason them away with facts.
   <u>Fact 1</u>: *"I have had A1Cs like this before and my endocrinologist has never called me lazy."*

Fact 2: *"I am not the only patient she sees with out-of-range numbers."*
Fact 3: *"Her job is to help me have better control, not discourage me. This is just an opportunity for her to show how great she is at her job."*

2) Replace them with positive thoughts.
    Affirmations are pre-rehearsed, positive thoughts we repeat to shift our thinking. They are short, sweet, and entirely up to you. For example:

"I take good care of myself."
"I will not worry about things out of my control."
"One more thing, one more time." -Josh Sundquist
"Every good decision improves my control."
"I am surrounded by people who want me to be my healthiest."
"These times may be difficult, but they are passing."
"I have many blessings." *Bonus if you name three

Affirmations can sound silly at times, but they are effective: it's impossible to hold onto negative thoughts when repeating positive words. Even in the absence of negative thoughts, repeating affirmations can help our mental strength throughout the day. Putting an affirmation in a place it can be seen regularly is a great way to take a proactively-positive view in the way we think about T1D.

Practicing Gratitude

In preparation for the Boston Marathon, I completed 80 training runs for a total of ~540 miles over the course of 20 weeks. And that's not counting the additional hundreds of miles worth of "pre-training" training from the six months prior. Or the thousands of miles that led to qualifying for Boston in the first place (and I'm on the lower end of mileage when it comes to distance runners!).

It goes without saying, but training for a marathon requires a lot of running. A lot of running over a long span of time. Not every training run is exciting. Truth be told, not many of them are. After awhile, training can seem mundane and check marks that runs equate to become commonplace. There are days when runners barely roll out of bed, complain about the weather, and pity themselves for feeling sore.

It takes change in the expected to take a step back. Events that interrupt routine running—sickness, injury, travel, etc.—serve as reminders that not a single run should be taken for granted…that the opportunity to run is a privilege. Nike sums this idea up perfectly in an old ad: "Running is a Gift." So powerful, yet so easy to forget.

What may seem like burdens of regular routine can actually be blessings in disguise. Going to school begets the opportunity to receive an education. Taking time to prepare meals allows us to be nourished. The never-ending string of training runs reflects having a healthy outlet for release. *T1D management gives us the chance to live.*

Yes, T1D management is rather annoying. We take shots…lots of shots. We go through enough test strips to build small, plastic villages. We count more carbs than the most religious of dieters. We endure literal highs and lows while balancing the highs and lows of life outside T1D.

But we have the opportunity to live. A blessing that not everyone gets to have. With many other conditions, there are no known treatments. Even for patients with T1D, treatment and even diagnosis can be impossible. Proximity to medical facilities is a barrier. Access to education and information is a barrier. Money is a barrier. In the not-so-distant past, every person with T1D lived without viable treatment. Rewind a little less than 100 years ago and insulin hadn't even been used to treat T1D! There are seniors in our nursing homes older than insulin therapy.

Countless discoveries, inventions, and advocacy efforts have transformed the way we live with T1D. From the very beginning, here are some of the most important innovations that created the understanding, treatments, and lifestyle we enjoy today:

~1,500 B.C.) Hesy-Ra, an Egyptian physician, recognizes frequent urination as a symptom in some of his patients. This account is thought to be the first mention of diabetes in history and is recorded on an Egyptian medical document called the Ebers Papyrus.

~400 B.C.) Physicians notice the urine of patients with diabetes is sweet in nature and attracts ants. To test for diabetes, physicians would instruct patients to urinate near an anthill. If ants congregated around the spot of urination, it indicated a positive diagnosis. The alternative diagnostic test was tasting urine to see if it contained sugar (ewww!).

17th century) Thomas Willis is the first to claim that diabetes is a disease of the blood. Before this time, physicians largely believed diabetes to be a disease of the kidneys and treatments focused mostly on alleviating excessive urination.

19th century) Claude Bernard hypothesizes that glucose is stored in the body. Bernard found that even during starvation, glucose remained in the bloodstream. He concluded that blood glucose must also come from a source other than food. His theory was confirmed when he found a substance in the liver made up of modified glucose molecules. He called this substance "glycogen" and introduced the importance of the liver in diabetes.

1869) At the age of 22, Paul Langerhans discovers that the pancreas contains two types of cells. One of these types he observed was spread over the organ in small clusters. They were later named the "islets of Langerhans."

1910) Sir Edward Albert Sharpey-Schafer discovers a substance produced by the islets of Langerhans that he names "insulin." The name comes from the Latin "insula" (island) due to the clustered nature of the islets of Langerhans cells.

1921) Frederick Banting and his student assistant, Charles Best, find that injecting insulin into dogs with removed pancreases caused their blood sugars to go down and diabetes symptoms to disappear. One year later in 1922, Banting and Best use insulin to treat diabetes in 14-year-old, Leonard Thompson. Upon receiving insulin that the hospital physician described as "thick, brown muck," Thompson's blood sugars lowered and he regained weight back to his frail, 65 lb frame.[6]

1923) Eli Lilly and Company and Novo Nordisk begin mass-producing insulin for treatment. The first insulins were made from the pancreases of pigs and cows and contained many impurities. Because of these impurities, patients would often have reactions at injection sites. Impurities also caused different vials of insulin to have different strengths (i.e., 5 units with many impurities would be less potent than 5 units without impurities). This made injections risky and highly experimental. Socially, doctors were outraged by the idea of patients giving themselves injections without medical training.

1949) The ADA guides the production of standard syringes to reduce insulin dosing errors. These syringes were much more cumbersome than the type we use today. Needles were sharpened with a whetstone and twisted onto a glass cylinder. Both parts of the syringe were boiled between shots and it was not uncommon for them to break. This made for a very time-consuming, delicate process. Not to mention, the needles were relatively more expensive and the gauge was much larger and more painful.

1950) Hans Hagedorn and his research team develop neutral protamine Hagedorn (NPH) insulin. This insulin was the first form of longer-acting insulin (now called intermediate) and could be mixed with short-acting. This reduced the number of shots people with diabetes were required to take each day.

1963) Arnold Kadish designs the first insulin pump. This pump was about the size of a backpack and was originally designed to deliver both insulin and glucagon. It would still take around 15 years to develop a more realistic model for patient use.

1970) The Ames Company produces the first blood glucose meter. Because blood glucose meters were so large (~3 lbs) and expensive (~$650 in 1970...the equivalent of over $4,000 in 2017),[7] they were only first available in hospitals and clinics. However, this gave a much more accurate estimate of real-time blood glucose than urine samples. Because urine tests could only detect sugar in the urine (which isn't present unless a patient exceeds the renal threshold for glucose ~180 mg/dL (10 mmol/L)), it was not helpful for monitoring in-range or low blood sugars.

1972) Insulin concentration becomes standardized at U100 (100 units/ml). Before, insulin was produced at different concentrations, requiring different dosing depending on the concentration used. With a standard insulin concentration, dosing errors decreased.

1977) Scientists develop the A1C test to measure the percent of glycosylated red blood cells. This was the first reliable indicator of blood sugar control over time and has since been used to guide research, recommendations, and treatment goals.

1980) The basal/bolus regimen is introduced as a treatment for T1D. Although it required more daily injections, this system allowed patients to have tighter control and more flexible lifestyles. Insulin could now be adjusted for daily changes in food and physical activity.

1981) Home glucose meters hit the market for patient use. With at-home meters, people with T1D could now have multiple blood glucose readings a day versus 3-4 times a year at doctor's visits. They were more informed in daily treatment decisions and were also provided extra protection with the ability to detect hypoglycemia prior to symptoms.

1982) The U.S. Food and Drug Administration (FDA) approves genetically engineered human insulin. Instead of relying on animal pancreases, injected insulins could now be of human origin and produced in a laboratory. This eliminated impurities and unpleasant reactions that still occasionally occurred at injection sites.

1983) Wearable insulin pumps are introduced for patient use. Before pumps evolved into the sleek types we use today, they were much bulkier and patients had more restrictions, including staying connected at all times...even for showers!

1986) Insulin pens are introduced for treatment. Instead of carrying around vials of insulin and syringes, supplies were now more centralized and portable. Drawing up the correct insulin doses also became more convenient, further reducing dosing errors.

1990) The Americans with Disabilities Act is passed, which prohibits discrimination based on conditions like T1D. Before, people who took insulin could suffer discrimination in the workplace due to the potential liability that comes with high and low blood sugars. Because of this, many people hid their T1D from their supervisors and coworkers. After this act was signed into law, people with T1D could be more open about management and have increased workplace awareness in the event of an emergency.

1993) The DCCT gives tangible data to show that tighter blood sugar control decreases chances of developing long-term complications. Importantly, this study showed that any period of improved control, even in a history of someone with a relatively higher A1C, produced better long-term outcomes.

1996) Insulin analogs are introduced, becoming the fastest and most predictable insulin on the market. Previously, the fastest insulin took 2-3 hours to peak and 3-6 hours to finish working versus insulin analogs that take 1-2 hours to peak and 3-4 hours to finish working.

1999) Virginia passes the first Safe at School law to ensure safety and fair treatment for students with T1D. Now, more than half of all states have similar laws that require training for school teachers and staff on how to care for students with T1D.

1999) The FDA approves the first CGM system. Similar to blood glucose meters, CGMs were first used only in clinics and hospitals to give more tailored treatment recommendations. It wasn't until 2006 that the first CGMs were approved for patient use. This gave people with T1D the power to see real-time trends, providing earlier indications of out-of-range numbers.

2001) Stem cells are found to have insulin-producing capabilities. Now, the mission continues to create a sustainable supply of stem cells that can be engineered to act like beta cells and avoid destruction by the body's immune system.

2013) The California Supreme Court rules in favor of giving non-medical, trained school personnel the ability to administer insulin to young students with T1D. This ruling ensured that students with T1D would have access to the insulin and supplies they need while at school, even in the absence of a school nurse.

2016) The FDA approves the first closed-loop insulin pump/CGM system for people with T1D. Using CGM monitoring, this system automatically adjusts the amount of basal insulin the user receives to increase time spent in range.

The opportunity to live a high-quality life with T1D is one that we are privileged to have…it's a gift, and we should never forget that.

Purpose

I got hooked on running marathons for a number of reasons. The feeling of accomplishment. The medals. The extra peanut butter. But the most compelling reason for running marathons is that it gives my life a greater sense of purpose. When I run, I'm not just running for myself—I am running for *all* people with T1D and those who believe in me. I am a representative. A role model. With every run, I prove that people with T1D are capable of accomplishing <u>anything</u>. These thoughts are often what gets me past the miles where I want to give up.

The lives we are able to live now with T1D are from the contributions of those who came before us. The people who devoted their lives to studying T1D and who participated in research, even during highly experimental times. The ones who advocated for our rights and made the general public more aware of T1D. And their work isn't finished. The day we were diagnosed with T1D, we became part of this legacy that is so much greater than ourselves. By continuing the work of those before us, we make a lasting impact on people living with T1D both right now and in the future. Everyone can offer unique gifts and experiences that do just that.

One of the easiest and most meaningful ways to continue this legacy is by participating in research. Studies range from surveys about our daily routines with T1D to clinical trials for cutting-edge treatments. They are located across the country and usually come with incentives such as money or free medical services. Each study is voluntary (i.e., you can choose to drop out at any time) and undergoes strict review by the Institutional Review Board to ensure participant safety. Once data is collected, it is used for <u>years</u> to inform those working toward better treatments and patient care. The National Institutes of Health has a full listing of all registered studies at clinicaltrials.gov, listed in Resources.

Another way to give back is by getting involved in the T1D community. Just as we use others' experiences and advice to become better in our own management, we can use our experiences and advice to guide others. We can be the emotional support someone needs during a rough time. The person who lets others know that they're not alone in the struggles they face.

Opportunities to be involved in the T1D community include national organizations such as JDRF, school clubs, summer camps, support groups (such as those offered through local hospitals), and online communities. Examples can be found in Resources.

With involvement in organizations devoted to creating better lives for people with T1D, there also comes opportunities to participate in advocacy events. These events raise money for research, help those who don't have access to treatment, inform policy makers, and educate the general public about the truths of T1D.

Of course if you find a real passion for T1D research, mentoring, or advocacy, you can make it a career! The increased understanding of scientists, health professionals, and policy makers who have T1D themselves or personal connections to T1D allows for invaluable insight and a profound impact in the T1D community.

By default, we were given purpose that some people search their entire lives to find. Having the power to relate to others on a deep level and change their lives is a blessing that should never be taken for granted. Every day, this purpose gives us the potential to *keep moving forward.*

A PERSONAL BEST

After crossing the finish line at 26.2 miles, a person takes on the title of "marathoner." That title is for life. It allows entry into a very special group of people and provides reassurance for every other challenge...*if I can run a marathon, I can do just about anything.*

Living with T1D shapes us in more ways than we can imagine. With diagnosis, we joined some of the bravest, most inspiring people in the world. We are set apart with the confidence that handling the challenges T1D throws our way conditions us to handle anything. To accomplish anything. To be afraid of nothing. In so many ways, T1D grants us the opportunity to be better people and leave an incredible mark on this world.

That mark is amplified by being the healthiest, happiest versions of ourselves we can possibly be. To pursue what we love doing most....live a life without limits. And better control is our enabler.

Just as marathon runners don't work to have "perfect" times, the only thing we work for in T1D is our *personal best.* Accepting no less than our best allows us to go beyond the limits we set for ourselves. It focuses on the journey and not the end result. With the right approach, our efforts accumulate to get us farther than we could ever imagine.

Growing up, my dad regularly repeated two pieces of advice:

"You only get one opportunity to make the most of today."

"Take care of the little pieces and the big picture will fall into place."

Every day's management matters and creates a little piece to our big picture. Every small step gets us closer to the place we want to be and the time to start training is now. Because in this life with T1D, we deserve nothing less than a personal best.

RESOURCES

Find an Expert

Academy of Nutrition and Dietetics
Eatright.org/find-an-expert
Find a local registered dietitian.

American Association of Clinical Endocrinologists
Aace.com/resources/find-an-endocrinologist
Find a local endocrinologist.

American Association of Diabetes Educators
Diabeteseducator.org/patient-resources/find-a-diabetes-educator
Find a local certified diabetes educator.

Integrated Diabetes Services
Integrateddiabetes.com
Staff of medical professionals with a focus on T1D management for athletes of all levels. Of special note, CDEs have T1D themselves and enjoy physical activity or participating in sports.

Nutrition and Physical Activity

Academy of Nutrition and Dietetics
Eatright.org
Nutrition, physical activity, and wellness tips tailored to specific populations (i.e., children, parents, men, women, and seniors).

American Council on Exercise
Acefitness.org/acefit
Fitness programs, workouts, tips for healthy living, recipes, and tools to find certified fitness professionals.

CalorieKing
Calorieking.com
App: CalorieKing Food Search
App and pocket-sized guides that contain nutritional information for over 70,000 foods and 260 restaurants.

Centers for Disease Control and Prevention
Cdc.gov/nutrition
Strategies for improving dietary quality and database of local programs.

Cdc.gov/physicalactivity
Strategies for increasing physical activity and database of local programs.

Office of Disease Prevention and Health Promotion, U.S. Department of Health and Human Services
Health.gov
Updated *Dietary Guidelines for Americans* and *Physical Activity Guidelines for Americans*.

U.S. Department of Agriculture
Choosemyplate.gov
Tips for nutrition, physical activity, and eating on a budget. "What's Cooking" tool offers recipes and menu planner.

University of Sydney
Glycemicindex.com
The most extensive database for GI values. Includes information about how GI values are determined, educational materials about using the GI in our care, and some of the latest nutritional research.

Continued Education Favorites

Books:

ADA Medical Management of Type 1 Diabetes by Francine Kaufman
A book written for medical professionals that explains the latest recommendations and gives a good idea of what doctors look for in managing our care. Updated every few years based on research outcomes.

Diabetic Athlete's Handbook: Your Guide to Peak Performance by Sheri Colberg
Breaks down the science of what happens physiologically during different types of exercise and offers guidance on finding strategies that work best for specific activities. Dr. Colberg makes complex concepts easy to understand.

Pumping Insulin by John Walsh and Ruth Roberts
John Walsh has used insulin pumps himself for over 30 years and combines his own experience with training as a Diabetes Clinical Specialist to offer a useful guide to effectively use insulin pumps. Used by both patients and physicians.

Think Like a Pancreas and *Until There Is a Cure* by Gary Scheiner
Gary Scheiner is a CDE with T1D. His writing is relatable and funny while including well-rounded information about T1D management. His books were among the first I read for continued education in college!

Publications (websites also feature many articles and resources):

A Sweet Life
Asweetlife.org
Articles on anything from nutritious recipes to the latest T1D public health research and everything in between.

Diabetes Forecast (published by the ADA)
Diabetesforecast.org
The ADA's publication that includes healthy recipes, technology reviews, research, advocacy initiatives, and inspiring stories of people with T1D.

Diabetes Health
Diabeteshealth.com
Articles on T1D care, community, healthy lifestyle, psychology, and celebrities with T1D as well as free apps for on-the-go learning.

Diabetes Self-Management (published by Rapaport Publishing)
Diabetesselfmanagement.com
Articles on diabetes management, recipes, and healthy lifestyle as well as additional resources for continued education.

Organizations:

American Diabetes Association
Diabetes.org/findaprogram
Database of local educational programs recognized by the ADA. Also offers free online learning programs.

Children with Diabetes
Childrenwithdiabetes.com
In-person conferences and online learning materials, including care suggestions backed by T1D research.

Integrated Diabetes Services
Integrateddiabetes.com
Website includes resources for checking insulin dosing, log templates, and newsletters for a summary of the latest diabetes updates.

JDRF (formerly the Juvenile Diabetes Research Foundation)
Jdrf.org
A comprehensive list of resources and research initiatives. Especially useful starting point for recently diagnosed people with T1D and their families.

Jewish Diabetes Association
Jewishdiabetes.org
Information on resources and research for everyone with T1D, but especially for those who balance management with Jewish customs.

Websites:

Diabetesdaily.com
Educational materials on everything from handling low blood sugars to starting a regular exercise routine. Great resources for those who are recently diagnosed. Also offers free in-person events.

Healthline.com/diabetesmine
Entries by patients and health professionals about advocacy initiatives, research, and treatments as well as interviews and guest posts from T1D celebrities.

Diabetesnet.com
Education on the essential tools for managing T1D and a comprehensive list of resources for further learning and involvement in the T1D community.

Diatribe.org
Columns on news, research, and advice as well as resources to help people with diabetes get the most from their therapies and lifestyle choices. Especially great for those who are recently diagnosed.

Insulinnation.com
Articles on lifestyle tips as well as the newest research and treatments in T1D. Articles also offered in Spanish.

Type1university.com
A wide range of free courses to sharpen management skills designed by CDEs.

Select Products and Applications

American Diabetes Association
Shopdiabetes.org
The ADA's online store that offers books, meal planning tools, and accessories for people with diabetes.

CalorieKing Food Search
Calorieking.com/foods
Contains nutritional information for over 70,000 foods and 260 restaurants.

Diabetes Pilot
Diabetespilot.com
Tracks blood sugars, medications, exercise, and nutritional information via an integrated database. Graphics help to find trends while reports can be shared with care team.

Diabetes 360
Diabetes360.deepbluewebtech.com
Bolus dose calculator based on individual insulin:carb ratios, correction factors, starting blood sugars, and carbohydrates. Linked to carbohydrate database from the USDA. Reports can be shared with care team.

Glooko
Glooko.com
Blood sugar and insulin pump data recorded manually or by synced app, nutritional information via an integrated database, logs for exercise that can link with fitness devices, and lifestyle notes to help find trends. Reports can be shared with care team.

Glucose Buddy
Glucosebuddy.com
Logs for blood sugars, insulin, food, and activity. Includes reminders for cues to remember management tasks. Visual reports to help find trends.

Inpen
Companionmedical.com/InPen
Insulin pen that links with smartphone to calculate bolus doses and track insulin action. Can program reminders into the app and share reports of insulin doses, carbohydrates, and blood sugars with care team.

PredictBGL
Managebgl.com
Bolus dose calculator, integration with fitness data, and logs for blood sugars and carbohydrates. Live data and report sharing with members of care team. Tools for mindfulness about unexpected highs and lows to help prevent them in the future.

MyFitnessPal
Myfitnesspal.com
Tracks exercise and nutrition while connecting users to a larger community of people who are also making efforts to be mindful of their lifestyle choices. Also great for accurate carb counting.

MySugr
Mysugr.com
Bolus dose calculator, synced or entered blood sugars, and visual reports. The mySugr scanner app allows users to scan blood sugars without syncing or cords.

One Drop Diabetes Management
Onedrop.today
Synced or entered blood sugars, physical activity, and insulin. Includes visual reports and an interactive community of people with diabetes.

Part III Templates
Everystepcountst1d.org
Website for the Every Step Counts Scholarship Program that recognizes healthy living with T1D, especially in young adults. Includes SMART template, log sheets, and charts for insulin:carb ratios and correction factors.

Road ID
Roadid.com
Customizable medical IDs that are easy to wear and great for an active lifestyle.

Timesulin
Timesulin.com
Cap over insulin pen that helps confirm dose amounts and how long ago doses were administered.

Involvement and Advocacy

American Diabetes Association
Diabetesstopshere.org
The ADA's blog featuring personal stories and the latest advocacy news.

Children with Diabetes
Childrenwithdiabetes.com
Conferences, online forums, and resources for youth and young adults with T1D as well as their parents and guardians.

College Diabetes Network
Collegediabetesnetwork.org
Information to help young adults balance T1D with college and professional careers. Provides opportunities for connection through local events and college chapters.

Diabetes Camping Association
Diabetescamps.org
Helps locate camps nationwide for people with diabetes to participate as campers or volunteers.

Beyond Type 1
Beyondtype1.org
An online community for people with T1D that offers information, news, and personal stories as well as programs for advocacy and connection such as a snail mail club and team that bikes across the country.

Tudiabetes.org
Beyond Type 1's outlet for people with T1D to talk about anything and everything T1D–mental and emotional wellness, food, treatments, diabetes technology, advocacy, and more.

International Diabetes Federation
Idf.org
Information about the global impact of diabetes and opportunities for international connection and advocacy.

Insulinforlife.org
Aids people who lack access to diabetes supplies such as those in low or middle-income countries and those who are victims of natural disasters.

JDRF (formerly the Juvenile Diabetes Research Foundation)
Jdrf.org
In-person and online resources for connection with others who have T1D and their families. Advocacy events offered nationally.

Typeonenation.org
JDRF's site to connect people with T1D through conversations, events, support teams, and tool kits for people with new diagnoses.

Jewish Diabetes Association
Jewishdiabetes.org
Connects Jewish people with T1D and discusses strategies that accommodate T1D care while maintaining Jewish customs.

MyGlu
Myglu.org
Partnered with the T1D Exchange to connect people with T1D while also offering opportunities to contribute our perspectives on the challenges of life with T1D and strategies we can use to improve our care.

Students with Diabetes
Studentswithdiabetes.com
Connects young adults with T1D on college campuses and within communities. Offers conferences, competitive internships, opportunities for advocacy, and resources to start new chapters.

Research

National Institutes of Health
Clinicaltrials.gov
The largest database for clinical trials in 195 countries. Search clinical trials by medical condition, location, and intervention for participation or to stay informed about the latest research.

TrialNet
Diabetestrialnet.org
T1D screening for relatives of people with T1D to research preservation of beta cell function and ultimately, preventing T1D in the future.

T1D Exchange
T1dexchange.org
Online research to advance quality of life for people with T1D. Open to both people with T1D and their families.

Scholarships and Awards

College Diabetes Network
Collegediabetesnetwork.org/content/scholarships
An extensive list of educational scholarships for young adults with T1D.

Eli Lilly and Company
Lillydiabetes.com/lilly-diabetes-journey-awards.aspx
Awards honor those who have lived 10, 25, 50, and 75 years with T1D.

Every Step Counts Scholarship Program
Everystepcountst1d.org
A college scholarship program I started in the fall of 2017 to recognize young adults for healthy living with T1D as they transition to fully independent care.

Joslin Diabetes Center
Joslin.org/joslin_medalist_program.html
Awards honor those who have lived 25, 50, and 75 years with T1D. Medalist Study explores factors that promote a long life of high quality in people with T1D.

ENDNOTES

Author's Note
1. Miller, K.M., et al., "Current state of type 1 diabetes treatment in the U.S.: Updated data from the T1D Exchange Clinic Registry," *Diabetes Care* 38 (2015), pp. 971-978.

Part I
1. American Diabetes Association, "Standards of medical care in diabetes—2017," *Diabetes Care* 40 (2017), pp. (Suppl. 1): S14-S80.
2. Estimated average glucose (eAG) to A1C conversion can be performed with the American Diabetes Association's eAG/A1C Converter online at: professional.diabetes.org/diapro/glucose_calc.
3. Fairbrother, N., *House in the Country* (New York: Knopf, 1965).
4. Scheiner, G.S., *Think Like a Pancreas* (Boston: Da Capo Press, 2011), pp. 14-18, 25-26.
5. Kaufman, F.R., *Medical Management of Type 1 Diabetes (6th ed.)* (Alexandria, VA: American Diabetes Association, 2012), p. 3.
6. Riebl, S.K. and Davy, B.M., "The hydration equation: Update on water balance and cognitive performance," *ACSM's Health and Fitness Journal* 17 (2013), pp. 21-28.
7. McEwan, B.S., "Central effects of stress hormones in health and disease: Understanding the protective and damaging effects of stress and stress mediators," *European Journal of Pharmacology* 583 (2008), pp. 174-185.
8. Powers, M.A., Richter, S.A., Ackard, D.M., and Craft, C., "Diabetes distress among persons with type 1 diabetes: Associations with disordered eating, depression, and other psychological health concerns," *The Diabetes Educator* 43 (2016), pp. 105-113.
9. The Diabetes Control and Complications Trial Research Group, "The effect of intensive treatment of diabetes on the development and progression of long-term complications in insulin-dependent diabetes mellitus," *The New England Journal of Medicine* 329 (1993), pp. 977-986.

10. Nathan, D.M. for the DCCT/EDIC Research Group, "The Diabetes Control and Complications Trial/Epidemiology of Diabetes Interventions and Complications Study at 30 years: Overview," *Diabetes Care* 37 (2014), pp. 1-16.
11. Galmer, A., *Diabetes (Biographies of Disease)* (Westport: Greenwood Press, 2008), p. 47.
12. Enzlin, P., Mathieu, C., Van Den Bruel, A., Vanderschueren, D., and Demyttenaere, K., "Prevalence and predictors of sexual dysfunction in patients with type 1 diabetes," *Diabetes Care* 26 (2003), pp. 409-414.
13. Kaufman, F.R., *Medical Management of Type 1 Diabetes (6th ed.)* (Alexandria, VA: American Diabetes Association, 2012), p. 253.
14. U.S. Department of Health and Human Services and U.S. Department of Agriculture, *2015-2020 Dietary Guidelines for Americans (8th Edition)* (2015). Available at: http://health.gov/dietaryguidelines/2015/guidelines/.
15. Colberg, S.R. and Edelman, S.V., *50 Secrets of the Longest Living People with Diabetes* (Boston: Da Capo Press, 2008), p. 147.
16. Herbst, A., Bachran, R., Kapellen, T., and Holl, R.W., "Effects of regular physical activity on control of glycemia in pediatric patients with type 1 diabetes mellitus," *Archives of Pediatric and Adolescent Medicine* 160 (2006), pp. 573-577.
17. Yip, J., Facchini, F.S., and Reaven, G.M., "Resistance to insulin-mediated glucose disposal as a predictor of cardiovascular disease," *The Journal of Clinical Endocrinology and Metabolism* 83 (1998), pp. 2773-2776.
18. U.S. Department of Health and Human Services, *2008 Physical Activity Guidelines for Americans* (2008). Available at: https://health.gov/paguidelines/guidelines/.

Part II

1. Longman, J., "Fastest marathon is run, but it's not a record," *The New York Times* 7 May 2017.
2. Joyner, M.J., "The marathon world record time is inching closer to 2 hours. Here's what it will take for a human to pass that threshold," *The Washington Post* 31 October 2014.
3. Joyner, M.J., "Modeling: optimal marathon performance on the basis of physiological factors," *Journal of Applied Physiology* 70 (1991), pp. 683-687.
4. Hutchinson, A., "An exclusive, behind-the-scenes look at how Nike is trying to break the 2-hour marathon barrier," *Runner's World* June 2017, pp. 62-73.

5. Tattersall, R., *Diabetes: The Biography (Biographies of Disease)* (Oxford: Oxford University Press, 2009), pp. 15-23.
6. Galmer, A., *Diabetes (Biographies of Disease)* (Westport: Greenwood Press, 2008), pp. 32-33.
7. Kaufman, F.R., *Medical Management of Type 1 Diabetes (6th ed.)* (Alexandria, VA: American Diabetes Association, 2012), p. 61.
8. American Diabetes Association, "Standards of medical care in diabetes—2017," *Diabetes Care* 40 (2017), p. (Suppl. 1): S49.
9. Coster, S., Gulliford, M.C., Seed, P.T., Powrie, J.K., and Swaminathan, R., "Monitoring blood glucose control in diabetes mellitus: a systematic review," *Health Technology Assessment* 4 (2000), pp. i-iv, 1-93.
10. Scheiner, G.S., *Think Like a Pancreas* (Boston: Da Capo Press, 2011), p. 169.
11. American Diabetes Association, "Standards of medical care in diabetes—2017," *Diabetes Care* 40 (2017), p. (Suppl. 1): S52.
12. Kaufman, F.R., *Medical Management of Type 1 Diabetes (6th ed.)* (Alexandria, VA: American Diabetes Association, 2012), p. 31.
13. Cobry, E., et al., "Timing of meal insulin boluses to achieve optimal postprandial glycemic control in patients with type 1 diabetes," *Diabetes Technology and Therapeutics* 12 (2010), pp. 173-177.
14. American Diabetes Association "Approaches to glycemic treatment," *Diabetes Care* 39 (2016), pp. (Suppl. 1): S52-S59.
15. Atkinson, F.S., Foster-Powell, K., and Brand-Miller, J.C. "International tables of Glycemic Index and Glycemic Load values," *Diabetes Care* 31 (2008), pp. 2281-2283.
16. Ibid.
17. Ibid.
18. Augustin L.S., et al., "Glycemic index, glycemic load, and glycemic response: An international scientific consensus summit from the International Carbohydrate Quality Consortium (ICQC)," *Nutrition, Metabolism, and Cardiovascular Diseases* 25 (2015), pp. 795-815.
19. Ibid.
20. Bondia, J., et al., "Coordinated basal-bolus infusion for tighter postprandial glucose control in insulin pump therapy," *Journal of Diabetes Science and Technology* 3 (2009), pp. 89-97.
21. Colberg, S.R., et al., "Physical activity/exercise and diabetes: A position statement of the American Diabetes Association," *Diabetes Care* 39 (2016), pp. 2065-2079.
22. American College of Sports Medicine, American Dietetic Association, and Dietitians of Canada, "Joint position statement: Nutrition and athletic

performance," *Medicine and Science in Sports and Exercise* 32 (2000), pp. 2130-2145.

23. Hacker Thompson, A., "Preventing the 'low-fuel light' in endurance exercise," *American College of Sports Medicine*, published online 7 October 2016. Available at: http://www.acsm.org/public-information/articles/2016/10/07/preventing-the-low-fuel-light-in-endurance-exercise.

24. Scheiner, G.S., *Think Like a Pancreas* (Boston: Da Capo Press, 2011), pp. 185-217.

Part III

1. U.S. Department of Health and Human Services and National Heart Lung and Blood Institute, *Your Guide to Healthy Sleep* (2005) NIH Publication No. 11-5271. Available at: https://www.nhlbi.nih.gov/files/docs/public/sleep/healthy_sleep.pdf.

2. Institute of Medicine of the National Academies, *Dietary Reference Intakes for Water, Potassium, Sodium, Chloride, and Sulfate* (Washington, D.C.: National Academies Press, 2005), p. 73.

3. Lally, P., van Jaarsveld, C.H.M., Potts, H.W.W., and Wardle, J., "How are habits formed: Modelling habit formation in the real world," *European Journal of Social Psychology* 40 (2010), pp. 998-1009.

4. Reese, R.J., "Just how bad is Heartbreak Hill?" *Runner's World*, published online 15 April 2013. Available at: http://www.runnersworld.com/run-the-numbers/is-the-boston-marathons-heartbreak-hill-as-bad-as-they-say.

Part IV

1. Taylor, N.S., "Cheer!" Old South Church: Blessing of The Athletes (Boston, MA) 19 April 2015. Available at: http://www.oldsouth.org/sermon/2015-04-19.

2. Petry, N.M., Cengiz, E., Wagner, J.A., Weyman, K., Tichy, E., and Tamborlane, W.V., "Testing for rewards: A pilot study to improve type 1 diabetes management in adolescents," *Diabetes Care* 38 (2015), pp. 1952-1954.

3. Berns, S., "My Philosophy for a Happy Life," *TEDx Mid-Atlantic Conference* (2013). Available at: https://ed.ted.com/on/Q0fBdrVh.

4. Scheiner, G., *Until There Is a Cure* (Ann Arbor, MI: Spry Publishing LLC, 2013), p. 131.

5. Dweck, C., "The Power of Believing That You Can Improve," *TEDxNorrkoping* (2014). Available at:

https://www.ted.com/talks/carol_dweck_the_power_of_believing_that_you_can_improve.

Dweck, C., M*indset: The New Psychology of Success* (New York: Ballantine Books, 2007).

6. Tattersall, R., *Diabetes: The Biography (Biographies of Disease)* (Oxford: Oxford University Press, 2009), p. 57.

7. Vaughn, R.A., *Beating the Odds* (Lexington, KY: CreateSpace Independent Publishing Platform, 2010), p. 109.

BIBLIOGRAPHY

American Diabetes Association "Approaches to glycemic treatment," *Diabetes Care* 39 (2016), pp. (Suppl. 1): S52-S59.

American Diabetes Association, "Standards of medical care in diabetes—2017," *Diabetes Care* 40 (2017), Suppl. 1.

American Diabetes Association, "75th Anniversary Timeline," (2014). Available at: http://www.diabetes.org/about-us/75th-anniversary/timeline.html.

Atkinson, F.S., Foster-Powell, K., and Brand-Miller, J.C., "International tables of Glycemic Index and Glycemic Load values," *Diabetes Care* 31 (2008), pp. 2281-2283.

Augustin L.S., et al., "Glycemic index, glycemic load, and glycemic response: An international scientific consensus summit from the International Carbohydrate Quality Consortium (ICQC)," *Nutrition, Metabolism, and Cardiovascular Diseases* 25 (2015), pp. 795-815.

Bell, K.J., Smart, C.E., Steil, G.M., Brand-Miller, J.C., King, B., and Wolpert, H.A., "Impact of fat, protein, and glycemic index on postprandial glucose control in type 1 diabetes: Implications for intensive diabetes management in the continuous glucose monitoring era," *Diabetes Care* 38 (2015), pp. 1008-1015.

Bertoluci, M.C., Cé, G.V., da Silva, A.M.V., Wainstein, M.V., Boff, W., and Puñales, M., "Endothelial dysfunction as a predictor of cardiovascular disease in type 1 diabetes," *World Journal of Diabetes* 6 (2015), pp. 679-692.

Bondia, J., et al., "Coordinated basal-bolus infusion for tighter postprandial glucose control in insulin pump therapy," *Journal of Diabetes Science and Technology* 3 (2009), pp. 89-97.

Cobry, E., et al., "Timing of meal insulin boluses to achieve optimal postprandial glycemic control in patients with type 1 diabetes," *Diabetes Technology and Therapeutics* 12 (2010), pp. 173-177.

Colberg, S.R., *Diabetic Athlete's Handbook* (Champaign, IL: Human Kinetics, 2009).

Colberg, S.R. and Edelman, S.V., *50 Secrets of the Longest Living People with Diabetes* (New York: Marlowe and Company, 2007).

Colberg, S.R., et al., "Physical activity/exercise and diabetes: A position statement of the American Diabetes Association," *Diabetes Care* 39 (2016), pp. 2065-2079.

Coster, S., Gulliford, M.C., Seed, P.T., Powrie, J.K., and Swaminathan, R., "Monitoring blood glucose control in diabetes mellitus: a systematic review," *Health Technology Assessment* 4 (2000), pp. i–iv, 1–93.

The Diabetes Control and Complications Trial Research Group, "The effect of intensive treatment of diabetes on the development and progression of long-term complications in insulin-dependent diabetes mellitus," *The New England Journal of Medicine* 329 (1993), pp. 977-986.

Enzlin, P., Mathieu, C., Van Den Bruel, A., Vanderschueren, D., and Demyttenaere, K., "Prevalence and predictors of sexual dysfunction in patients with type 1 diabetes," *Diabetes Care* 26 (2003), pp. 409-414.

Galmer, A., *Diabetes (Biographies of Disease)* (Westport: Greenwood Press, 2008).

Herbst, A., Bachran, R., Kapellen, T., and Holl, R.W., "Effects of regular physical activity on control of glycemia in pediatric patients with type 1 diabetes mellitus," *Archives of Pediatric and Adolescent Medicine* 160 (2006), pp. 573-577.

Lally, P., van Jaarsveld, C.H.M., Potts, H.W.W., and Wardle, J., "How are habits formed: Modelling habit formation in the real world," *European Journal of Social Psychology* 40 (2010), pp. 998-1009.

Lovett, C., *Olympic Marathon: A Centennial History of the Games' Most Storied Race* (Westport, CT: Praeger Publishers, 1997).

McEwan, B.S., "Central effects of stress hormones in health and disease: Understanding the protective and damaging effects of stress and stress mediators," *European Journal of Pharmacology* 583 (2008), pp. 174-185.

Nathan, D.M. for the DCCT/EDIC Research Group, "The Diabetes Control and Complications Trial/Epidemiology of Diabetes Interventions and Complications Study at 30 years: Overview," *Diabetes Care* 37 (2014), pp. 1-16.

Petry, N.M., Cengiz, E., Wagner, J.A., Weyman, K., Tichy, E., and Tamborlane, W.V., "Testing for rewards: A pilot study to improve type 1 diabetes management in adolescents," *Diabetes Care* 38 (2015), pp. 1952-1954.

Powers, M.A., Richter, S.A., Ackard, D.M., and Craft, C., "Diabetes distress among persons with type 1 diabetes: Associations with disordered eating, depression, and other psychological health concerns," *The Diabetes Educator* 43 (2016), pp. 105-113.

Riebl, S.K. and Davy, B.M., "The hydration equation: Update on water balance and cognitive performance," *ACSM's Health and Fitness Journal* 17 (2013), pp. 21-28.

Scheiner, G.S., *Think Like a Pancreas* (Boston: Da Capo Press, 2011).

Scheiner, G.S., *Until There Is a Cure* (Ann Arbor, MI: Spry Publishing LLC, 2013).

Tattersall, R., *Diabetes: The Biography (Biographies of Disease)* (Oxford: Oxford University Press, 2009).

U.S. Department of Health and Human Services, *2008 Physical Activity Guidelines for Americans* (2008). Available at: https://health.gov/paguidelines/guidelines/.

U.S. Department of Health and Human Services and U.S. Department of Agriculture, *2015-2020 Dietary Guidelines for Americans (8th Edition)* (2015). Available at: http://health.gov/dietaryguidelines/2015/guidelines/.

Vaughn, R.A., *Beating the Odds* (Lexington, KY: CreateSpace Independent Publishing Platform, 2010).

Walsh, J. and Roberts, R., *Pumping Insulin (5th ed.)* (San Diego: Torrey Pines Press, 2013).

Yip, J., Facchini, F.S., and Reaven, G.M., "Resistance to insulin-mediated glucose disposal as a predictor of cardiovascular disease," *The Journal of Clinical Endocrinology and Metabolism* 83 (1998), pp. 2773-2776.

ACKNOWLEDGMENTS

All glory to God for every breath, step, and experience—all of it belongs to You. I pray this book finds its way to those You know it will inspire. Thank You for Your strength and for the following people who have helped me in life with type 1 diabetes, running marathons, and the writing process:

My mom, who I will never be able to repay for her selflessness. You have woken up thousands of times in the middle of the night to test my blood sugar and without you, I wouldn't be alive. Thank you for always sharing in my dreams and helping to make them happen.

My dad, "Big Steve," who gives me countless words of wisdom every day (I hope you read this book long enough to see that some made it in near the very end). One day we will write a book with one piece of your advice on every page. And when we do, it'll be a novel and a half.

My sister, Brooke, who I look up to literally and figuratively. You make every room brighter when you walk in, yet underneath that gracious, fun-loving appearance is grit I can't even begin to describe. I am inspired by you and proud of all that you do in service to this country.

Thomas, who makes me a better person every day. None of this would have happened without you. You are my adventure and I can't wait to see where this life takes us.

Mrs. Moran, who I shared this project with in its earliest stages. You supported me every step of the way...even after I scrapped the entire first draft.

Erin and Isabel, who put up with me that year after college when all I did was write in our apartment, and then complain that I didn't like any of it. Despite those underwhelming testaments to my writing ability, you somehow still believed this project would come to completion. You both kept me going when I wanted to quit and I owe so much of this book to your encouragement.

The Konapelskys, who has been a second family to me since David and I met at the JDRF Night of Hope Gala in high school. Thank you for giving me a place to stay and always having my back!

My pediatric care team of Dr. Touchette, Dr. Cogen, and Celia who cared for me above and beyond what was expected. Your teamwork was indispensable to my health and inspired my future goal of becoming a doctor.

My undergraduate mentor, Ken, who still believes in me more than I do myself. I will always work to make you proud!

Dr. Ickes, who required me to write a draft of this book's outline upon graduation. It has changed a lot since May 2015, but you probably knew at the time that it would. Thank you for telling me to go for it.

My mentors at the NIH, Dr. Chen and Dr. Cypess, who taught me to be a better thinker and communicator. Because of you, I have a critical eye for all work, but mostly my own. I strive to emulate both of you as I pursue a career in medicine and research.

Win, who finds genuine appreciation for everyone around him. Your life is an inspiration and sitting next to you at the liver talk could not have been more serendipitous.

Rose, who graciously went over this manuscript amidst a move to Australia. Your ability to converse about anything and everything is beyond impressive and your considerate nature is even more so.

Gary Scheiner and Dr. Sheri Colberg, who have been long-time inspirations to me in the T1D community and advised me in the writing process. Your expertise has been invaluable to my learning and I look forward to working with you in the future.

Finally, my friends and colleagues with T1D who inspire me every day, especially: Caity, David, George, Patrick, Emily, Kristin, Delia, Alex, Elliot, Gaby, Gracie, Ramón, Katarina, Caitlin, Alexi, Erik, Phil, Devin, Aaron, and Trish. Last but not least, the inspiration for this book: Linda.

Printed in Poland
by Amazon Fulfillment
Poland Sp. z o.o., Wrocław